Surgical Technique of the Abdominal Organ Procurement

Andrzej Baranski

Surgical Technique of the Abdominal Organ Procurement

Step by Step

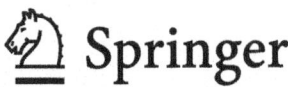 Springer

Andrzej Baranski, MD, PhD
Department of Surgery and Organ Transplantation
Leiden University Medical Centre
Leiden
The Netherlands

ISBN: 978-1-4471-6207-0   ISBN: 978-1-84800-251-7 (eBook)
DOI: 10.1007/978-1-84800-251-7

British Library Cataloguing in Publication Data
© Springer-Verlag London Limited 2009
Softcover re-print of the Hardcover 1st edition 2009
Apart from any fair dealing for the purposes of research or private study, or criticism or review, as permitted under the Copyright, Designs and Patents Act 1988, this publication may only be reproduced, stored or transmitted, in any form or by any means, with the prior permission in writing of the publishers, or in the case of reprographic reproduction in accordance with the terms of licences issued by the Copyright Licensing Agency. Enquiries concerning reproduction outside those terms should be sent to the publishers.
The use of registered names, trademarks, etc. in this publication does not imply, even in the absence of a specific statement, that such names are exempt from the relevant laws and regulations and therefore free for general use.
Product liability: The publisher can give no guarantee for information about drug dosage and application thereof contained in this book. In every individual case the respective user must check its accuracy by consulting other pharmaceutical literature.

9 8 7 6 5 4 3 2 1

springer.com

This book is dedicated to the following people who have been – and are still – important in my life:

Prof. Dr. J. Nielubowicz (1915–2000), Prof. Dr. J. K. Szmidt, Prof. Dr. J. Polanski, S. Frunze: my surgery teachers from Warsaw University Medical School, Warsaw, Poland who taught and guided me during my first steps in surgery.

W.S.L. Kowalski, BChD, LDSRCS (Eng), MA who, for many years, has been both a friend and a sounding board whom I trust and respect.

Prof. Dr. J.H. van Bockel from Leiden University Medical Centre, Leiden, The Netherlands, who has inspired me to write this book.

Finally, I want to express my respect, thanks and love to my wife, Ewa Anna Baranska Szczepanowska, my daughters Katarzyna and Julia, my parents, Zofia and Bernard, and my parents-in-law Wieslawa and Jan Szczepanowscy – my dearest, who always love and believe in me.

Preface

The intention of this book is to promote a surgical technique of abdominal organ procurement in order to avoid organ damage and thus enhance the quality of retrieved organs.

Organ procurement from a brain death donor is an essential part of organ transplantation. In donors where more than one organ is removed, the surgical procedure is critically important and could be challenging both for the procurement and recipient surgeons. Surgical injury or inadequate preservation of organs at this stage may cause irreversible organ damage or can lead to serious complications in the recipient.

Nowadays, local or regional surgical teams, whereby the transplant surgeon is not always one of the team members, perform most multiorgan donor (MOD) procurement procedures. To trust each other and to avoid surgical mistakes, adequate training and standardization of the surgical techniques is required. Teaching and training future procurement surgeons to adopt a standard operating procedure could be the right way to prevent technical mistakes and damage during abdominal multiorgan procurement.

I hope that in the near future, every transplant surgeon involved in organ procurement will have to be certified. The different national and international transplant organizations in Europe have been already started to establish the teaching programs, which will lead to high expertise in the field of abdominal organ procurement.

My personal view is to recommend mandatory registration of the quality of procured organs by the national transplant organizations and that this data should be published both in the interest of the transplant community and in the interest of the public who have a right to this information.

I wish to help every reader to experience the pleasure and satisfaction of successful multiorgan procurement.

Leiden, May 9th 2008   Andrzej G. Baranski

Contents

Introduction xv

1 Transplant Coordinator–Procurement Team: Bilateral Aid and Understanding, Before, During and After Abdominal Organ Procurement 1

    1.1 Introduction 1
    1.2 The Services of the Donor Coordinator 2
    1.3 The Most Important Moments of Communication: Priority of Interests 3
        1.3.1 Before Organ Procurement 3
        1.3.2 During Organ Procurement 5
        1.3.3 After Organ Procurement 6
    1.4 Conclusion 7
    Literature 8

2 Preoperative Arrangements for Organ Donation 9

    2.1 Donor Preoperative Arrangements 9
        2.1.1 Arrival of the Abdominal Procurement Team at the Donor Hospital 9
        2.1.2 Donor Verification 12
        2.1.3 Positioning Donor on the Operating Table 13
        2.1.4 Shaving 14
        2.1.5 Scrubbing 15
        2.1.6 Draping: Covering the Body with Sterile Operating Sheets and Incision Drapes 17
        2.1.7 Installation of the Abdominal Retractor 19
    Literature 20

3 Incision and Exposure 21

    3.1 Abdominal and Thoracic Incision 21
        3.1.1 Abdominal Incision 21
        3.1.2 Median Sternotomy 26

		3.1.3	Wide, Stable Thoracic and Abdomen Operating Field: The Retractors	30
	Literature			32

4 Detailed and Thorough Abdominal Organ Inspection 33

- 4.1 Introduction 33
- 4.2 Liver 34
  - 4.2.1 General Examination 34
  - 4.2.2 Size of the Liver 34
  - 4.2.3 Parenchyma Inspection with Respect to Micro and Macrosteatosis 35
  - 4.2.4 Examination of Arterial Blood Supply to the Liver 36
- 4.3 The Pancreas 39
  - 4.3.1 Routes for Surgical Access 39
  - 4.3.2 Pancreas Inspection – Organ Assessment 42
- 4.4 Inspection of Other Abdominal Organs 43
  - 4.4.1 Gut Inspection 43
  - 4.4.2 Additional Investigations During Organ Inspection 43
- Literature 44

5 Retroperitoneal Right-Sided Visceral Mobilisation: The Cattel–Braasch Manoeuvre 45

- 5.1 Introduction 45
- 5.2 Right Colon Mobilisation 46
  - 5.2.1 Surgical Steps 46
- 5.3 Extended Kocher Manoeuvre – Duodenopancreatic Mobilisation ... 48
  - 5.3.1 Surgical Steps 48
- 5.4 Small Bowel Mobilisation 51
  - 5.4.1 Surgical Steps 51
- Literature 53

6 Infrarenal and Superior Mesenteric Artery Major Vessel Dissection 55

- 6.1 Abdominal Aorta and Inferior Vena Cava 55
  - 6.1.1 Surgical Steps 55
- 6.2 Superior Mesenteric Artery 64
  - 6.2.1 Surgical Steps 64
- Literature 64

7 Left Liver Lobe and Supraceliac Aorta 65

- 7.1 Preparation 65
  - 7.1.1 Colon and Small Bowel 65
- 7.2 Left Liver Lobe Mobilisation 66

	7.2.1	Surgical Steps	66
7.3	Visualisation of the Abdominal Aorta Beneath the Diaphragm		72
	7.3.1	Surgical Steps	72
7.4	Right Liver Lobe		74
	7.4.1	Surgical Steps	74

8 Hepatoduodenal Ligament and Biliary Tree ... 75

8.1	Definition, Ligament Inspection and Dissection		75
	8.1.1	Definition	75
	8.1.2	Hepatoduodenal Ligament Inspection: In Steps	76
8.2	The Common Bile Duct (CBD) Dissection		79
	8.2.1	Surgical Steps	79
8.3	The Gallbladder		81
	8.3.1	Possibilities of Treatment: In Steps	81
8.4	Right Aberrant Hepatic Artery		84
	8.4.1	Anatomy of the Aberrant Hepatic Artery	84
8.5	Gastroduodenal and Hepatic Artery Dissection		84
	8.5.1	Surgical Steps	84
8.6	Portal Vein – Dissection		86
	8.6.1	Surgical Steps	86
Literature			87

9 Small Bowel ... 89

9.1	Introduction		89
9.2	Small Bowel Dissection		90
	9.2.1	Surgical Steps	90
Literature			91

10 Thorax Procurement Team(s) ... 93

10.1	Abdominal Organ Protection		93
	10.1.1	Tip	93
	10.1.2	Dissection of the Thoracic Organs in Sequence	95
	10.1.3	An Arrangement with the Thorax Procurement Team(s) About the Following	95

11 Preparation for Organ Perfusion ... 97

11.1	Preservation Solution		97
	11.1.1	What Is Your Choice UW Or HTK, Or Celsior Preservation Solution?	97
	11.1.2	Storage	98

	11.2 Abdominal Aorta Perfusion System	99
	11.2.1 Preparation Technique in Steps	99
	11.3 Inferior Vena Cava Decompression System	101
	11.3.1 Preparation Technique	101

12 Major Abdominal Vessel Cannulation 103

   12.1 Agreement 103
      12.1.1 Communication Skills 103
   12.2 Ligation and Cannulation of the Abdominal Aorta and IVC 104
      12.2.1 Surgical Steps 104

13 Cold Perfusion 111

   13.1 Start Thoracic Organ Perfusion 111
      13.1.1 Introduction 111
   13.2 Start Abdominal Organ Perfusion 113
      13.2.1 Introduction 113
      13.2.2 Clamp Removal 114
      13.2.3 Topical Cooling 115
      13.2.4 Check Efficiency of the Abdominal Organ Perfusion System 116
   Literature 118

14 Thoracic Organ Procurement 119

   14.1 Introduction 119
      14.1.1 Sequence of Abdominal Organ Procurement 120
   Literature 123

15 Sequence of Abdominal Organ Procurement 125

   15.1 Small Bowel Procurement 126
      15.1.1 Surgical Steps 126
   15.2 Pancreas, Liver, Kidneys Procurement Surgical Technique 126
      15.2.1 Introduction 126
      15.2.2 Sterilizing Duodenum Content 128
      15.2.3 Dividing Duodenum from the Stomach 130
      15.2.4 Stomach Mobilisation 132
      15.2.5 Placing Small Bowel and the Colon Outside the Abdomen 136
   15.3 Pancreas and Liver Vascular Splitting 143
      15.3.1 Surgical Steps 143
      15.3.2 Pancreas Procurement 149
      15.3.3 Cutting SMA with Aortic Patch: In Steps 156

		15.3.4	Whole Pancreas Procurement for Islets Isolation: Surgical Technique	157
		15.3.5	Summary	159
	15.4	Liver Procurement		159
		15.4.1	Surgical Steps	159
	15.5	Kidney Procurement		169
		15.5.1	Separately: Surgical Steps	169
		15.5.2	En Block Kidney Procurement: Surgical Steps	178
		15.5.3	Separation of Kidneys Procured En Block in Steps	180
	Literature			183
16	**The Toolkit**			185
	16.1	Important Tool During the Transplantation Process		185
		16.1.1	Composition	185
		16.1.2	Surgical Technique of Toolkit Procurement and Packing	187
17	**Organ Packing**			189
	17.1	Technique of Organ Packing		189
		17.1.1	Introduction	189
		17.1.2	Organ Packing in Steps	190
		17.1.3	Kravitz's Lifeport Kidney Transporter	194
	Literature			194
18	**Post-Procurement Care of the Donor Body**			195
	18.1	Before Closing the Donor Body		195
		18.1.1	Surgical Steps	195
	18.2	Closing		195
		18.2.1	Surgical Steps	195
		18.2.2	Wound Dressing	198
19	**Operative Report and the Quality Forms**			199
	19.1	Organ Procurement is an Acknowledged Surgical Procedure		199
		19.1.1	Filling Reports	199
		19.1.2	Summation (Debriefing) of the Whole Procedure Together with the OR Personnel and TC	202
Index				203

Introduction

There are many ways to perform abdominal organ procurement (1–19). In this book, I describe the abdominal multiorgan procurement operation, which is performed on a hemodynamically stable, brain death donor. Brain death is defined as a complete, irreversible, and permanent cessation of electric activity of the brain, including the brain stem. The donor is defined as a heart-beating donor (HBD) (6).

Most organ donation for organ transplatation is done in the setting of a brain death, heart-beating donor (HBD).

The donor selection criteria are different for each organ and sometimes there are differences between the transplant centers. According to the literature (15–22), there are no more traditional limits concerning donor selection.

Generally, donor criteria in abdominal organ transplantation are as follows:

- Kidney from birth until 75 years
- Liver from first month until 70 years
- Pancreas from fifth year until 50–55 years
- Small bowel from 14th birthday or weight more than 3 kg until 50 years
- Multivisceral, according to the guidelines of the recipient center

The surgical technique of abdominal multiorgan procurement described here consists of 55–60% organ dissection and is performed with an intact donor circulation. I propose a technique in which time-consuming preparations have been limited to the anatomical landmarks. The necessary dissection is reduced to the minimum to split the abdominal organs with the main goal of preventing vascular and parenchymal abdominal organ damage.

The most important reason to perform organ retrieval in this way is both to reduce the cold ischemia time to a minimum and to avoid potential injury from extended ex-vivo manipulations. In-situ abdominal organ separation promotes direct organ sharing among centres through direct shipment from the donor hospital (20, 21).

Surgeons and surgical residents participating in organ procurement teams, who wish to quickly learn about abdominal organ procurement, as well as experienced surgeons who wish to refresh their knowledge just before abdominal organ donation will be the main beneficiaries of this book.

All photographs of the surgical steps in multiorgan abdominal procurement published in this book have, since 2000, been annually presented during the

National Courses on the Abdominal Multi Organ Donation organized by the National Dutch Transplant Foundation and Leiden University Medical Centre, Leiden, The Netherlands. In 2002, some of the figures and the photographs were published on a CD ROM entitled "Abdominal Multiorgan Donation Procedure" supported by an unrestricted educational grant from Fujisawa GmbH, now Astellas. At this point in my book, I want to express my special thanks to Mr. Albert Groenewoud, European Brand Director – Transplantation, Astellas Pharma Europe for interest in and promotion of abdominal multiorgan donation in Europe. In 2004, the European Society for Organ Transplantation (ESOT) took the initiative to include this course as a part of the education program (www.esot.org). Since 2005, this material has been presented during the annual international European Donor Surgery Masterclass (EDSM) course in Leiden University Medical Centre, Leiden, The Netherlands.

Literature

1. Rosenthal JT, Shaw BJ Jr, Hardesty RL, et al (1983) Principles of multiple organ procurement from cadaver donors. Ann Surg: 198: 617–621
2. Starzl TE, Miller C, Broznick B, Makowka L (1987) An improved technique for multiple organ harvesting. Surg Gynecol Obstet: 165: 343–348
3. Nghiem DD, Schulak JA, Corry RJ (1987) Doudenopancreatectomy for transplantation. Arch Surg: 122: 1201–1206
4. Marsh CL, Perkins JD, Sutherland DER, et al (1989) Combined hepatic and pancreaticoduodenal procurement for transplantation. Surg Gynecol Obstet: 168: 254–258
5. Wright FH, Smith JL, BowersVD, et al (1989) Combined retrieval of liver and pancreas grafts: alternatives for organ procurement. Transplant Proc: 21: 3522
6. Cooper DK, Novitzky D, Wicomb WN (1989) The pathophysiological effects of brain death on potential donor organs, with particular reference to the heart. Ann R Coll Surg Engl: 71: 261–266
7. Sollinger HW, Vernon WB, D'Alessandro AM, et al (1989) Combined liver and pancreas procurement with Belzer-UW solution. Surgery: 106: 685–690
8. Stratta RJ, Taylor RJ, Spees EK, et al (1991) Refinements in cadaveric pancreas–kidney procurement and preservation. Transplant Proc: 23: 2320–2322
9. Shaffer D, Lewis WD, Jenkins RL, et al. Combined liver and whole pancreas procurement in donors with a replaced right hepatic artery. Surg Gynecol Obstet 1992; 175: 204–207
10. Nakazato PZ, Concepcion W, Bry W, Limm W, Tokunaga Y, Itasaka H, et al. Total abdominal evisceration: an en bloc technique for abdominal organ harvesting. Surgery 1992; 111: 37–47
11. Shaffer D, Lewis WD, Jenkins RL, Monaco AP (1992) Combined liver and whole pancreas procurement in donors with a replaced right hepatic artery. Surg Gynecol Obstet: 175: 204–207
12. de Ville de Goyet J, Hausleithner V, Malaise J, et al (1994) Liver procurement without in situ portal perfusion: a safe procedure for more flexible multiple organ harvesting. Transplantation: 57: 1328–1332
13. de Ville de Goyet J, Reding R, Hausleithner V, et al (1995) Standardized quick en bloc technique for procurement of cadaveric liver grafts for pediatric liver transplantation. Transpl Int: 8: 280–285

14. Sindhi R, Fox IJ, Heffron T, et al (1995) Procurement and preparation of human isolated small intestinal grafts for transplantation. Transplantation: 60: 771–773.
15. Squifflet JP (1995) A quick technique for en bloc liver and pancreas procurement. Transpl Int: 9: 520–521
16. Imagawa DK, Olthoff KM, Yersiz H, et al (1996) Rapid en bloc technique for pancreas-liver procurement. Improved early liver function. Transplantation: 61: 1605–1609
17. Nghiem DD (1996) Rapid exenteration for multiorgan harvesting: a new technique for the unstable donor. Transpl Proc: 28: 256–257
18. Pinna AD, Dodson FS, Smith CV, et al (1997) Rapid en bloc technique for liver and pancreas procurement. Transpl Proc: 29: 647–648
19. Abu-Elmagd K, Fung J, Bueno J, et al (2000) Logistics and technique for procurement of intestinal, pancreatic, and hepatic grafts from the same donor. Ann Surg: 232: 680–687
20. Jan D, Renz JF (2005) Donor selection and procurement of multivisceral and isolated intestinal allografts. Curr Opin Organ Transpl: 10:136–147
21. Molmenti EE, Molmenti P, Molmenti H, et al (2001) Cannulation of the aorta in organ donors with infrarenal pathologies. Dig Dis Sci: 46: 2457–2459

Chapter 1
Transplant Coordinator–Procurement Team: Bilateral Aid and Understanding, Before, During and After Abdominal Organ Procurement[1]

Abstract Background: Organ procurement is the lifeblood of organ transplantation. A tense competitive atmosphere in the operating room (OR) and unprofessional communication skills between transplant coordinator (TC) and the members of organ retrieval team(s) may lead to inadequate preservation or surgical injury to the organs. At this stage, all mistakes, which have been made, can make an organ unsuitable for transplantation either due to impossible surgical reconstruction or because of damage – leading to serious complications in the recipient.

Successful communication means that you have to fulfil the following criteria: be responsive, engaging, pleasant, patient, clear, positive, realistic, and a problem solver. In the OR never criticize anyone in front of others; if you do so, it will probably cause your colleague to *lose face* but you will lose the respect of those who view the incident. Focus your criticism on the task and not on the person. This applies to the surgeon as well as the TC.

Conclusion: Organ donation procedure is more than *just go and get organs*. It is an essential part of the organ transplantation and contributes for at least 50% to its success or failure.

Keywords Transplant coordinator, Procurement team, Organ procurement, Communication skills

1.1 Introduction

Organ procurement is the lifeblood of organ transplantation (1, 2). A tense, competitive atmosphere in the operating room and/or unprofessional communication skills between the members of organ retrieval team(s) may lead to inadequate

---

[1] Fragments in this chapter have been published earlier in the following article: Baranski AG (2006) Transplant coordinator–procurement surgeon bilateral aid and understanding, before, during, and after organ procurement. Organs, Tissues and Cells, 3, 195–198.

preservation or surgical injury to the organs. At this stage, all mistakes, which have been made, can make an organ unsuitable for transplantation or they can lead to serious complications in the recipient.

The first formal organ procurement organization (OPO) was the New England Organ Bank in USA founded in 1968. This OPO and the 57 others across the United States were founded "as medical communities recognized the need to establish organizations that could expedite the procurement, preservation and distribution of organs" (1, 2).

The first transplant coordinator in Europe was appointed in the UK in 1979 based upon the idea that originated in the United States (5). Most of the TC(s) have responsibility for both organ donation and transplantation.

In some countries this role has been split up for procurement (donor) and recipient transplant coordinators both providing a 24 h service for their specialities (4, 5).

1.2 The Services of the Donor Coordinator

- Identification and selection of the potential donor
- Review and procurement of the appropriate and prescribed medical, legal and social consent from donor family
- Support and advice surrounding donor care in intensive care unit (ICU)
- Evaluation of the potential risk for the recipient
- Arrangement of the practical procedures involving the anaesthetist, the organ retrieval operation and sometimes pathologist, bacteriologist and radiologist support as well as the donor ICU
- Coordination of land/air transportation for the procurement team
- Support of the medical and nursing staff in the operating theatre throughout the process of procurement of the spleen and lymph nodes, up to, and including, the packaging and labelling of specimens
- Delivery of blood and tissue specimens to laboratories after the removal of the organs
- Distribution of donated organs to the appropriate transplant acceptor centres
- Logistics concerning the return (repatriation) of the retrieval team
- Advice and support to families before and after donation
- Feedback to the family, donor hospital staff and to the organ retrieval team(s) (2, 3, 4, 5, 6, 7)

During the whole process of organ procurement both the surgeon and the TC have to communicate regularly not only with each other, but also with many other people who are present in the OR. Coordination in such a multifaceted procedure requires high communication skills between people of different status, levels of competence and sex, in order to avoid misunderstandings, errors and medical mistakes (8, 9).

There are no standard instructions, nor is there any literature regarding the rules as to how the TC should communicate with the surgeon and the rest of the medical staff before, during and after organ procurement.

There is also no interactive training available for the surgeons to teach them how they should communicate with the transplant coordinator and other people before, during and after organ harvesting in order to achieve an optimal team spirit and to avoid quarrels, medical errors, misunderstandings and scandals.

1.3 The Most Important Moments of Communication: Priority of Interests

Communication between the TC and the surgeon during organ retrieval can be broken down into the following segments:

- Before – the initial contact and transportation to the donor hospital
- During – preparation for – and performance of – the operation
- After – paper work, discussion, feedback and support for the family and the medical staff

1.3.1 Before Organ Procurement

The first phone call to the procurement surgeon has to be done after initial assessment of the donor by the coordinator when the authorization of the organ removal has been obtained.

What the donor surgeon should hear and/or should discuss with the TC during the first contact, in most of the cases by telephone are as follows:

- Greeting and introduction
- In which hospital/country she/he is
- Age, weight, height of the donor and the recipients
- Reason for brain death or withdrawal of treatment
- State and treatment of the donor (stable or not)
- Whether the patient has been confirmed or not as having the clinical criteria for brain death or whether withdrawal of treatment is envisaged
- All potential risks for the recipient and for the procurement team (infectious disease, surgical operations, usual and unusual medication and treatments)
- Which organs have been accepted (heart, lungs, liver, pancreas, small bowel, kidneys)
- Kind of procedure – heart-beating donor (HBD) or non-heart-beating donor (NHBD)

- Approximate time of departure and type of transportation (land/air) to the donor hospital
- Distance and destination (whether a passport will be necessary or not)
- Time schedule for the procurement of organ(s)
- Medical equipment in the donor hospital (retractors, sterile ice, sterile cold fluids, povidone–iodine 2% in water solution, staplers, organ preservation solutions, operating theatre clothing, magnification glasses, sterile organ bags, sterile ice, coolbox, antibiotics, steroids, invasive monitoring equipment, etc.
- The required instruments that the procurement team must bring to the donor hospital (4, 5, 6, 7, 8)

A proverb says: If you fail to plan, you plan to fail. To indicate how such difficulties can arise, I will give you an example of a conversation between a TC and the surgeon, which I have witnessed. This is a typical example of complete misunderstanding of the role of the coordinator at the beginning of organ retrieval:

TC:	Good evening,
Surgeon:	Good evening, who is speaking?
TC:	Doctor – wake up, you have to leave your home, in 10 min an ambulance will pick you up. I will see you soon, bye.
Surgeon:	But....
TC:	Doctor – are you on duty?
Surgeon:	Yes, who are you? What time is it now?
TC:	Wake up. There is an ambulance waiting for you in front of your home. Hurry up, you have to fly tonight
Surgeon:	But who is speaking?
TC:	The TC, I must finish, now, I am very busy, I'll see you later, bye

After such a communication, I guarantee that the procurement surgeon, after arrival at the donor hospital, will not be able to create a warm, friendly, and close working relationship with the transplant coordinator.

In principle, the task of the TC is to safely coordinate land/air transportation of the procurement team to the donor hospital (4, 6, 7).

During transportation to the donor hospital, just in case of donor deterioration, the TC has to keep contact and inform the donor and the recipient surgeon. If necessary, the TC has to arrange the quickest means of transportation for the procurement team to the donor hospital.

In case of a cardiac arrest, the TC has to ask the local surgeon to perform major vessel cannulation and to start organ perfusion and cooling. The TC, if necessary, has to facilitate contact between the local and procurement surgeons in case of limited experience.

1.3.1.1 Preparation for the Operation in the Donor Hospital

Generally, the first thing, which has to be done, is to establish a good collegial relationship with the medical staff and the OR community:

1.3 The Most Important Moments of Communication: Priority of Interests

- The TC is waiting for the team at the agreed appointed place
- The procurement team alights from the ambulance and they introduce themselves to their host
- The TC brings the procurement team to the changing room
- The TC introduces the procurement team to the OR assistants, anaesthesiologist and local transplant coordinators, OR personnel and the other procurement teams

The surgeon, together with the TC, should have enough time to explain and discuss the surgical technique planned with the OR nurses and choose the necessary surgical instruments. During the explanation, be sure to remember that organ retrieval has a huge emotional impact on the OR personnel (9, 10, 11).

During donor evaluation *trust no one*. As a procurement surgeon, personally, together with the TC, verify and evaluate all information over the donor identity, age, weight, length, ABO compatibility with the recipient, confirmed clinical criteria of brain death, authorisation for the removal of organs (objectives) or authorisation for the withdrawal of treatment. Remember that, as often as not, the TC has a reputation for being busy and tired and may therefore forget to pass on important information about the donor (e.g. 3 years ago a patient had a very serious accident and underwent four abdominal operations and the sodium 1 h ago was 190, but that does not matter, all organs have been accepted) (11).

One more time, personally and together with the TC, analyse the past history of the patient: surgical operations, usual and unusual medication and/or treatments, danger or increased risk to the procurement and operating room personnel due to an infectious disease (HIV, HCV).

The TC has to report to the procurement surgeon as to which organs have to be retrieved and which of them have been accepted. Further, he/she should inform the surgeon about the donor family and recipient surgeon's wishes and the operation time schedule. The possibility of a quick intra-operative diagnosis is also very important to achieve the final product – a well-procured organ – and then to transplant it into the body of the recipient.

1.3.2 During Organ Procurement

At this time maximal coordination and cooperation between the TC and the procurement surgeon is required. The main goal of organ procurement is to minimize warm ischemic time and the efficient, rapid and safe removal of all accepted, usable organs for transplantation.

1.3.2.1 Duties of the Procurement Surgeons

The procurement surgeon must do the following:

- Inform the TC and everyone in the operating theatre that he/she is ready to start cold perfusion.

- Inform the TC about the state of organ perfusion and how many litres of preservation solution he/she will want to use and to check the quality of organ perfusion; if necessary replace or reposition aorta's cannula.
- Communicate with the TC about the wishes of the family and the recipient surgeon (toolkit).

1.3.2.2 End of Organ Procurement

- All organs have to be packed according to the National or Eurotransplant regulations; if the surgeon has to do this, the TC has to let him/her know.
- The TC has to inform every organ recipient centre when unexpected circumstances arise.

1.3.3 After Organ Procurement

Before departure, the surgeon should ensure that all necessary paper work has been completed. This work should be done together with the TC. A summary of the procedure should be worked out with the OR personnel. The procurement surgeon has to be the leader of pleasant debriefing about what went well, what went wrong and what could be done better the next time.

After the organs have been donated and retrieved, the TC should give feedback to the donor family and the procurement team.

To avoid medical mistakes and errors the most important thing for everyone involved in the organ procurement process to adopt is a proper, clear, adequate, and honest attitude, on the same level of communication with each other.

Good communication and a correct collegial behaviour between the people involved in the organ procurement plays the largest role in the avoidance of dangerous consequences for the organ recipients and/or for the medical staff.

Lingard et al. (5) found that 31% of all OR communications could be categorised as a failure. One of the key reasons for miscommunication arises from frictional power relationships, which exist in healthcare, because of different professional groups with a traditionally different status, and of a culture where hierarchy still resembles a military model.

Gudykunst (10) has described how misunderstandings arise during conversations between people of different status and sex because of their very different ways of communicating and expectations – for example, to demonstrate their status on the one hand, or to show their solidarity with colleagues on the other. Expectations involve our anticipations and predictions about how strangers will communicate with us. Our expectations are derived from social norms, communication rules and strangers' characteristics of which we are aware.

During organ procurement, everyone who is involved has to communicate adequately. There is also place for criticism. Successful communication means that you have to fulfil the following criteria: be responsive, engaging, pleasant, patient, clear, positive, realistic, and a problem solver (8). In the OR never criticize anyone in front of others. If you do so, it may cause the targeted person to *lose face* but what is even more important, you will lose the respect of those who have seen the incident. Focus your criticism on the task and not on the person. This applies to the surgeon as well as the TC.

1.4 Conclusion

I will now summarize the most important moments at which the procurement surgeon and the TC must be in harmony and communicate with each other on the same level of confidence.

They must be in agreement as to the following:

- The start of the operation
- The result of the abdominal organ inspection (tumour, injury, infection)
- The quality of the organs accepted for transplantation
- The need of additional examinations such as open or needle biopsy, ultrasonography, quick bacteriological and pathological examination
- The final judgment as to which organs are suitable for transplantation
- The vascular anatomy of the accepted organs, and who must inform the acceptor centre
- The sterilization of the duodenum content during pancreas procurement
- With the other procurement teams and TCs about donor heparinization, time of major vessel cannulation, preservation solutions and use of unusual medicines
- Allowing the other teams to prepare thoracic organs

If you want to feel good and respected, try to communicate properly; if it is impossible, just follow a course in communication.

Bilateral aid and understanding between the transplant coordinator and the surgeon before, during and after organ procurement could have a huge influence on the team spirit and the quality of the procured organs. Remember that the consequences of your poor communication skills will ricochet not just on the recipient, but also upon yourself (11).

Together with the TC and the procurement team you represent the transplant community.

Multi-organ donation procedure is more than *just go and get organs*. It is an essential part of organ transplantation and contributes for at least 50% to the success or failure of the result (2, 5, 10, 11).

Literature

1. Monteo TD (2002) The business of organ procurement. Current Opinion in Organ Transplantation, 7, 60-64
2. Manson RH (1993) Uniform Anatomical Gift Act. Statutory Regulation of Organ Donation in The United States, 2nd edition, South Eastern Organ Procurement Foundation, Richmond, VA
3. Kirkman RL, Mitford EL, Luskin RS (1993) The New England Organ Bank—lessons from running a regional bank. In: Terasaki PI, Cecka JM, eds. Clinical Transplants 1993. Los Angeles, CA: UCLA Tissue Typing Laboratory, 317–24
4. Lopez-Navidad A, Domingo P, Viedma MA (1997) Professional characteristic of the transplant coordinator. Transplantation Proceeding, 29, 1607-1613
5. López-Navidad A, Caballero F, Domingo P, Esperalba J, Viedma MA (1999) Hospital professionalization of the organ procurement process maximizes the retrieval potential. Transplant Proceeding, 31:1039-1039
6. Falvey S (1996) The role of the transplant coordinator. The Journal of the Royal Society of Medicine, 89 (Suppl 29), 18
7. British Transplantation Society (2003), Standards for Solid Organ Transplantation in the United Kingdom, 2nd edition, British Transplantation Society (ed), Triangle House, UK, pp. 15-17
8. Mosacula C, Arevallilo S, Cano T et al (2003) The nurse role in the Spanish model. Transplantation Proceeding, 35, 990-991
9. Awad SS, Fagan SP, Bellows C, De La Garza M, Berger DH et al. (2005) Bridging the communication gap in the operating room with medical team training. The American Journal of Surgery, 190, 770-774
10. Lingard L, Espin S, Whyte S et al. (2004) Communication failures in the operating room: an observational classification of recurrent types and effects. Quality and Safety in Health Care, 13, 330-334
11. Gudykunst WB (1998) Bridging Differences, Effective Inter-group Communication, 3rd edition, Sage, London.
12. Kuo P (2000) Organs In an Imperfect World Unexpected Donor Circumstances at St. Elsewhere, Duke University Medical Centre, Durham, NC
13. Denny R (2006) Communicate to Win, 2nd edition, Kogan Page, London, pp. 34-74

Chapter 2
Preoperative Arrangements for Organ Donation

Abstract Background: Having arrived at the donor hospital, the procurement team has to observe a prescribed protocol in organ procurement. First, the transplant coordinator (TC) should introduce the surgeons to the operating room personnel. One of the surgeons has to check, together with scrub nurse(s), the readiness of the operating room (OR) and explain the operating technique. In the meantime, the senior surgeon verifies the donor chart together with the transplant coordinator. Realization of all the above named tasks will allow transfer of the donor from ICU to the OR, to move him onto the operating table, and to start all preoperative preparations such a positioning, shaving, scrubbing, draping, and abdominal retractor installation.

Conclusion: A pleasant working atmosphere, good planning, professionalism, and finally very good communication skills between the OR members who are involved in organ procurement are necessary to avoid friction, quarrels, misunderstandings, and medical mistakes before and during preoperative arrangements for multiorgan procurement.

Keywords Donor verification, Donor shaving, Scrubbing, Draping, Abdominal retractor, Procurement team, Donor arrangements

2.1 Donor Preoperative Arrangements

2.1.1 Arrival of the Abdominal Procurement Team at the Donor Hospital

1. The procurement team is introduced by the transplant coordinator to the anaesthesiology team, scrub nurses, and the OR personnel (Fig. 2.1).
2. One of the procurement surgeons together with the scrub nurse(s) checks the operating room (OR) for the following:

    (a) General cleanliness and readiness (Fig. 2.2)

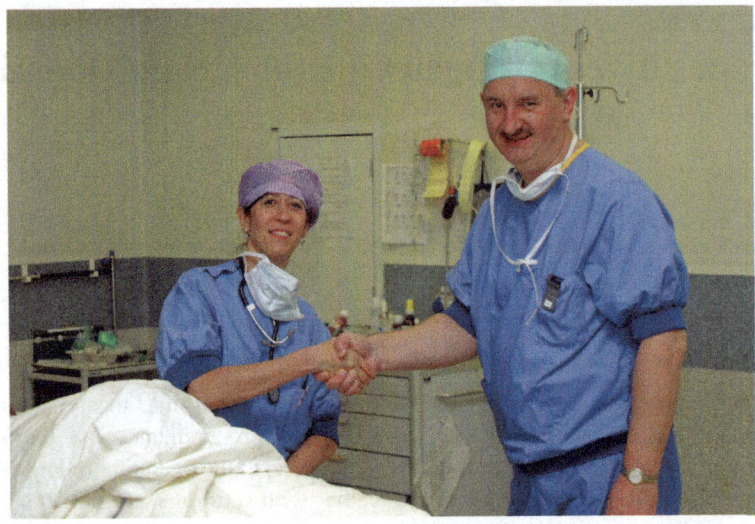

Fig. 2.1 Procurement team is introduced by the transplant coordinator to the anaesthesiology team, scrub nurses, and OR personnel

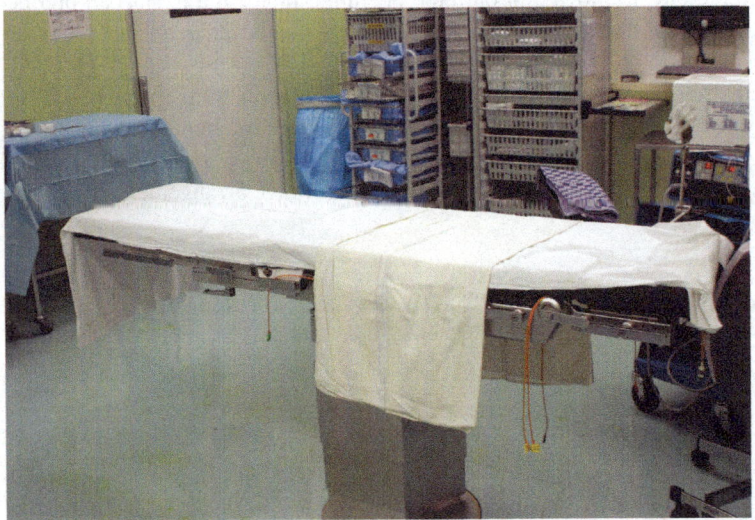

Fig. 2.2 General cleanliness and readiness – operating room inspection

(b) Presence of the required surgical equipment in good working order. The most important are as follows:

   i. Good functioning suction system (Fig. 2.3a)
   ii. Professional abdominal and thoracic retractors (Fig. 2.3b)

2.1 Donor Preoperative Arrangements

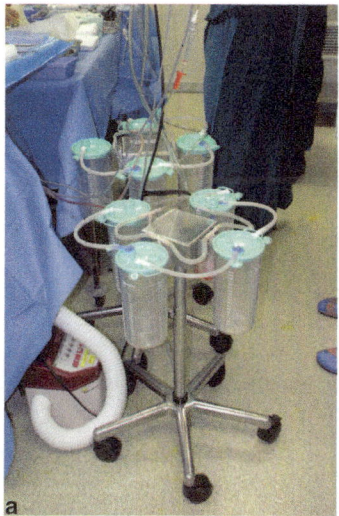

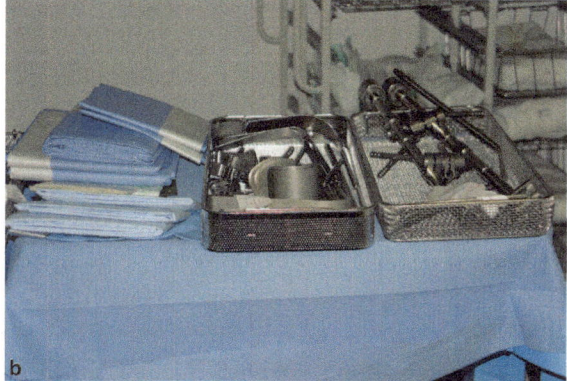

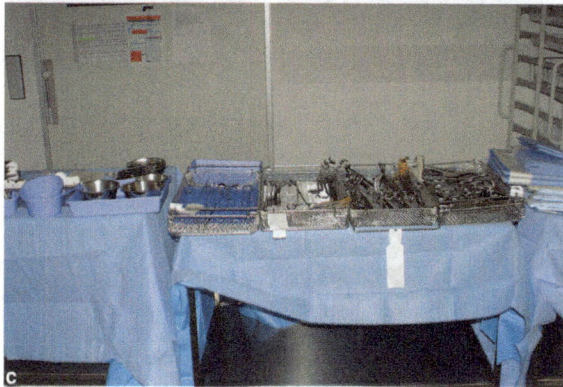

Fig. 2.3 Necessary surgical equipment – **a** good, functioning, professional suction system, **b** Necessary surgical equipment – professional retractor, **c** Necessary surgical equipment – surgical instruments

iii. Necessary instruments (Fig. 2.3c)
   iv. Drains, sternal saw, etc.

ATTENTION!
If you want to feel good and respected during operation explain to the OR personnel about the most important steps of the operation, including listing of the organs accepted for procurement and transplantation.

2.1.2 Donor Verification

1. Check, one more time, together with the transplant coordinator the patient's chart and verify the following:

    (a) Donor identity
    (b) Statement of brain death
    (c) Donor codicil
    (d) Medical history, ensure that it is complete and in order (Fig. 2.4)

2. In exceptional situations, the surgeon assists the transfer of the patient from ICU to the operating room (OR).

ATTENTION!
There is a quite high possibility of encountering the donor family at the donor's bedside in the ICU. Consequently, the ICU seems to me not the best place for the procurement surgeon at the beginning of the procedure.

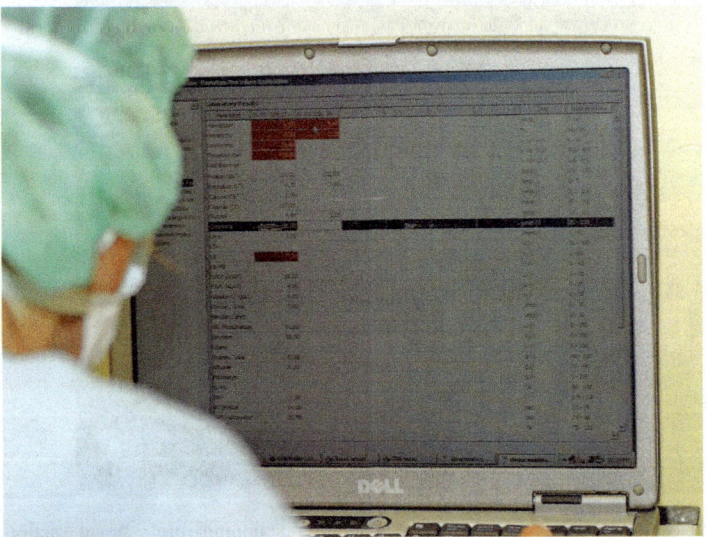

Fig. 2.4 Check one more time, together with transplant coordinator, the patient's chart and verify his/her identity

2.1 Donor Preoperative Arrangements

Remember that the family could react in a very emotional way when the procurement surgeon is present in the ICU.

2.1.3 Positioning Donor on the Operating Table

1. Try to obtain optimal exposure of the neck, thorax, and the abdomen.
2. Place the donor in the supine position (*on the back*):
   (a) Both arms are abducted 80; on boards (Fig. 2.5).
   (b) Legs should lie flat and uncrossed
3. The neck is extended by placing a sandbag under the shoulders (as during tracheotomy or thyroid surgery) (Fig. 2.6a).
4. Patient's eyelids should be carefully closed and taped to avoid corneal abrasion and dehydration. Direct pressure on the eye should be avoided; ensure that no part of the breathing equipment is pressing on the patient's face (Fig. 2.7).
5. During positioning, perform a brief medical examination with regard to skin cancer, postoperative scars, wounds, haematomas, deformations, slight and grievous body injury, etc.

ATTENTION!
All information resulting from the medical investigation performed during organ procurement could be very important and useful for police and justice departments especially during mandatory investigation.

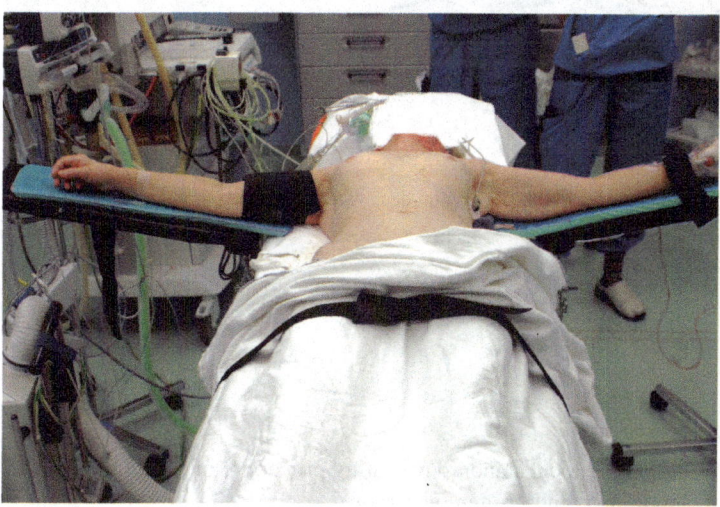

Fig. 2.5 Donor positioned on the operation table

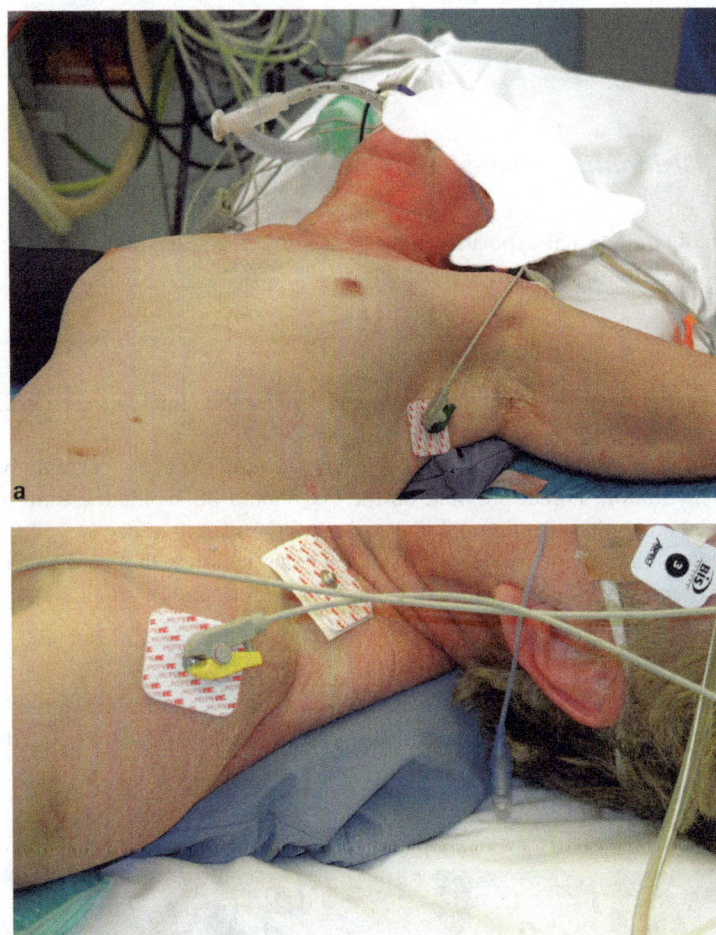

Fig. 2.6 **a** Neck extension, **b** Closing in, neck extension sandbag under the shoulders

2.1.4 Shaving

1. According to the local standard operating procedure of the donor hospital (neck, thorax, abdomen, and urogenital region).
2. During shaving, avoid damaging the donor skin – use a mechanical shaver (Fig. 2.8).

2.1 Donor Preoperative Arrangements

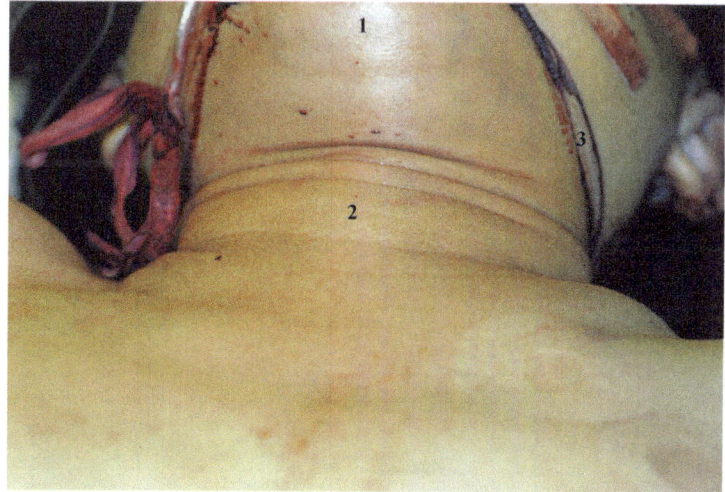

Fig. 2.7 Bandage fixing the endotracheal tube is pressing on the patient's face. 1 – Chin, 2 – Neck, 3 – Bandage

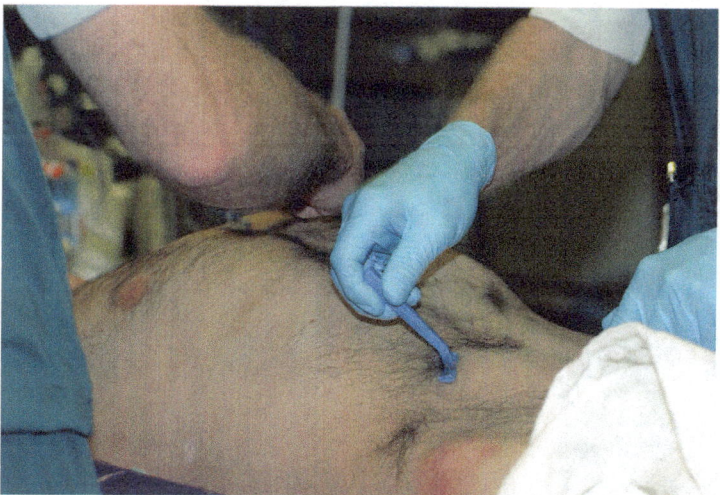

Fig. 2.8 Shaving – according to the local SOP (standard operating procedure); try to avoid damage to the skin

2.1.5 Scrubbing

1. The surgical team or the scrub nurse may perform the scrubbing of the donor according to the local standard procedure (neck, thorax, abdomen, and urogenital region) (Fig. 2.9).

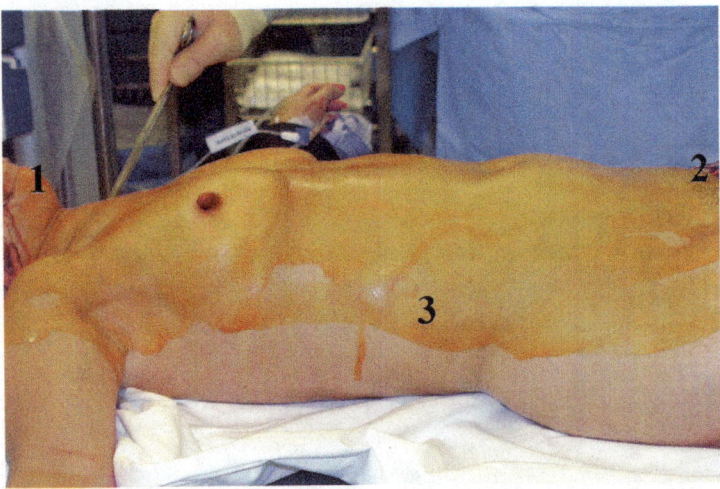

Fig. 2.9 Donor scrubbing – neck, thorax, abdomen, and urogenital region have been disinfected. 1 – Chin, 2 – Os pubis, 3 – Auxillary line

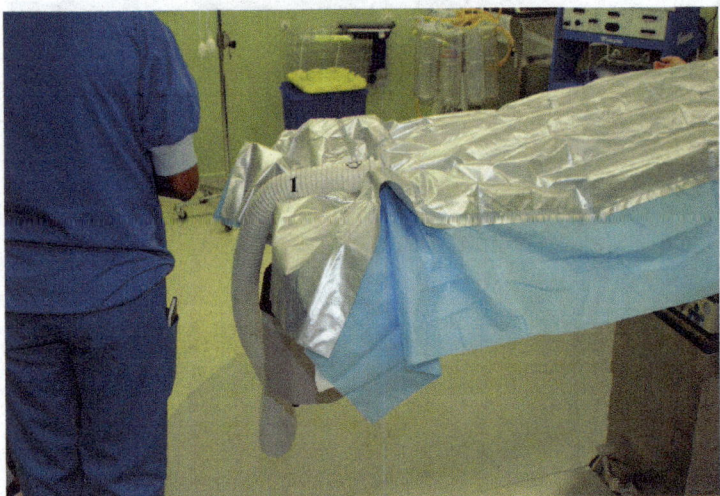

Fig. 2.10 Warm the donor body both before and during the whole multiorgan procurement procedure to avoid coagulation problems. 1 – Professional operating room warming system

ATTENTION!
- Do not use allergic or irritating skin substances for disinfection.
- Before disinfection always ask about possible donor allergy.
- Allergic shock is not a good sign at the beginning of organ procurement.
- Warm the donor body during the whole organ procurement procedure to avoid coagulation problems (Fig. 2.10).

2.1 Donor Preoperative Arrangements

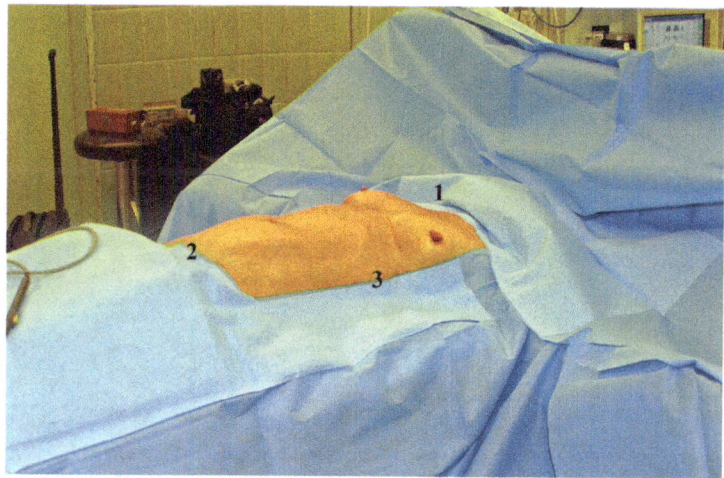

Fig. 2.11 The body is covered with sterile sheets: 1 - 3 cm above incision of manubrium sterni, 2 - 1–2 cm under the lever of the symphysis, 3- both sides until anterior auxillary line

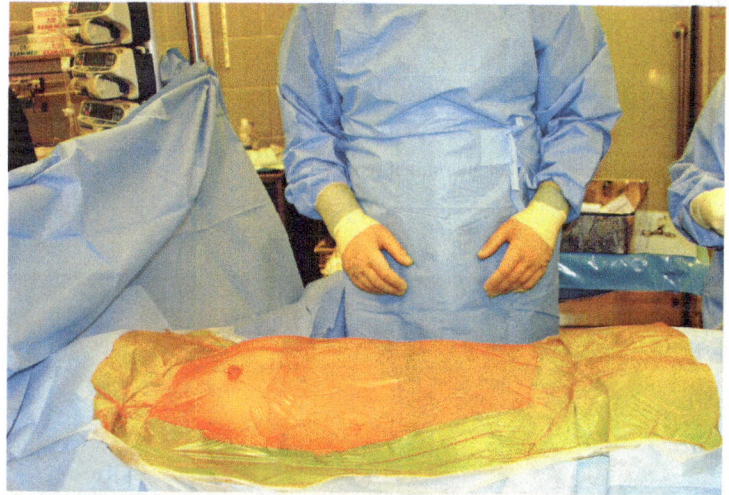

Fig. 2.12 Operating field is covered with an antimicrobial incision drape: Steri-Drape Ioban (3M)

2.1.6 Draping: Covering the Body with Sterile Operating Sheets and (Fig. 2.11) Incision Drapes

1. Proximal about 3 cm above incision of the manubrium sterni
2. Distal about 1–2 cm under the level of the symphysis
3. Lateral on both sides until anterior auxiliary line

4. Draping – covering the operating field with sterile incision drape Steri-Drape Ioban (3M) (Fig. 2.12)

ATTENTION!
- Always use steri-drape; it is critical to help reduce and restrict microorganisms from entering the open surgical wound (1, 2).

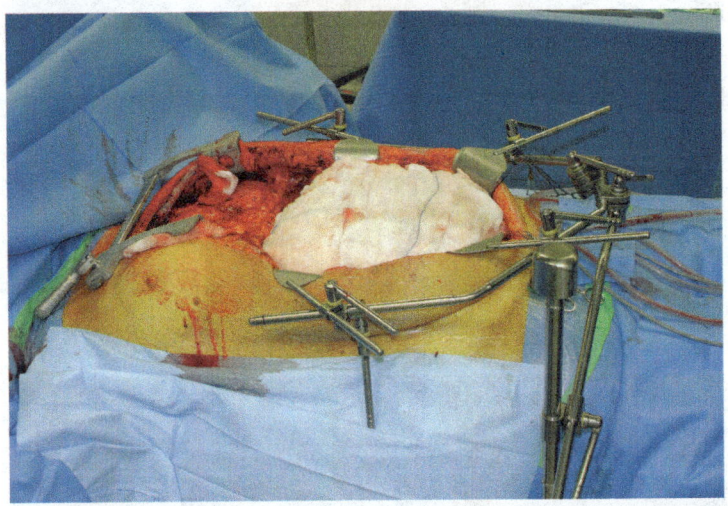

Fig. 2.13 OmniTrack professional abdominal retractor in use

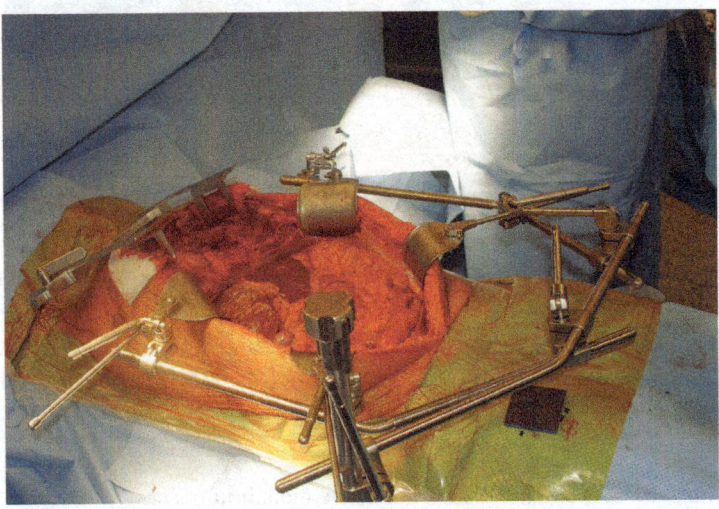

Fig. 2.14 Thompson professional abdominal retractor in use

2.1 Donor Preoperative Arrangements

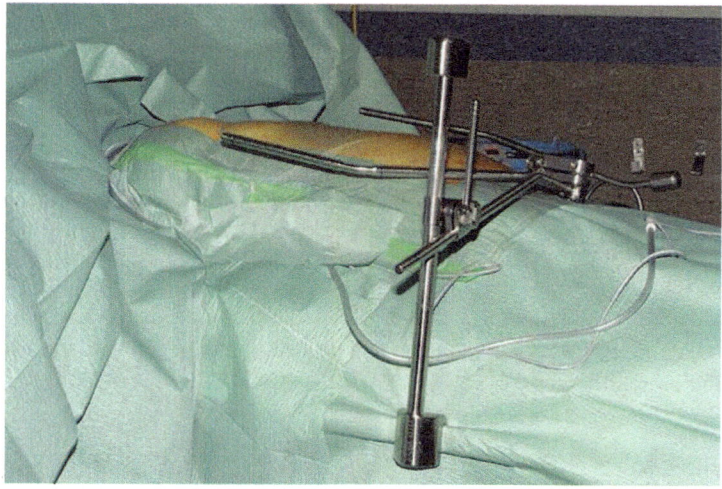

Fig. 2.15 Sterile post is placed on the operating table rail 8–10 cm below the os pubis and secured

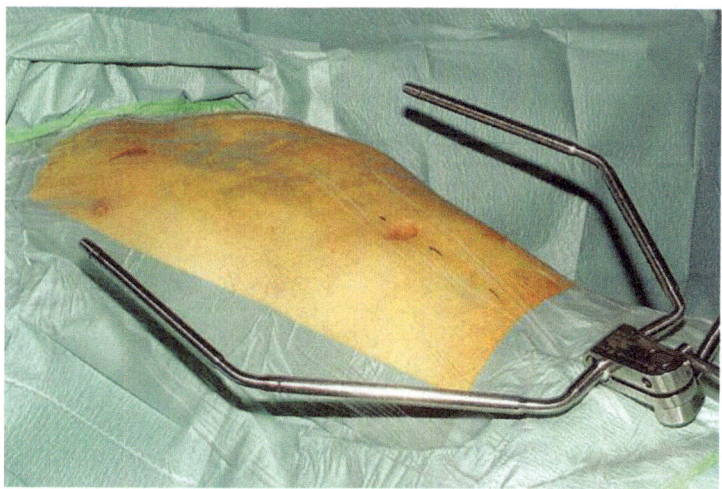

Fig. 2.16 The arms of the abdominal retractor are adjusted, secured, spread, and turned toward the donor's head

2.1.7 Installation of the Abdominal Retractor

1. Introduction: Use the abdominal retractor or a retraction system that is very flexible and in addition, allows retraction in all four directions. At the Leiden University Medical Centre, during different teaching courses, I always instruct

people in the use of one of two types abdominal retractors: Omni Track® from OminiTrack Surgical (Fig. 2.13) or Thompson® from Thompson Surgical Instruments Inc. (Fig. 2.14) during the multiorgan donation procedures (3, 4).
2. Place over the sterile drape post of the retractor and secure it onto the table rail 8–10 cm below of the os pubis (Fig. 2.15).
3. Adjust the wishbone (arms) of the abdominal retractor to the sterile post and secure it. The arms have to be spread, secured, and turned toward the donor's head (Fig. 2.16).

ATTENTION!
- A good abdominal retractor will provide you with a wide, stable operating field; it causes little or less organ damage, and ensures that you can work quicker, better, and more efficiently.

Literature

1. Guideline for Prevention of Surgical Site Infection, Center for Disease Control, U.S. Public Health Service, Revision 1999, Vol. 20, No. 4
2. 3MTM IobanTM 2 Antimicrobial Incise Drapes EZ from 3M. http://www.3M.com
3. Thompson Surgical Instruments Inc. http://www.thompsonsurgical.com
4. Omni – Trac Surgical. http://www.omni-tract.com

Chapter 3
Incision and Exposure

Abstract Background: A wide, stable operating field during abdominal multi-organ procurement is necessary to avoid abdominal organ injury. Thanks to the availability and use of professional abdominal and thorax retractors, an excellent approach to the thoracic and abdominal organs can be obtained. Wide, stable operating field means less risk for organ damage during its retrieval.

Particularly with the older donors (above 65 years old) with a higher chance of abdominal malignancy, it could be useful to perform a median laparotomy first, followed by a general abdominal organ inspection. If, after that, there are no contraindications for abdominal organ procurement, the second step sternotomy may be performed.

Conclusion: Wide, stable operating field can be achieved with the use of professional abdominal and thoracic retractors. With older donors with a higher chance of malignancy, it could be useful to perform a laparotomy first, followed by general abdominal organ inspection and sternotomy.

Keywords Abdominal incision, Sternotomy, Laparotomy, Abdominal retractor, Thoracic retractor

3.1 Abdominal and Thoracic Incision

3.1.1 Abdominal Incision

1. First perform an abdominal incision from the sternum xiphoid process to the os pubis (Fig. 3.1).
2. Cut and ligate (to avoid bleeding from the umbilical vein) teres ligament of the liver (Fig. 3.2).
3. Cut liver falciform ligament up to the hepatic veins close to the abdominal wall and the diaphragm (electrocautery) (Fig. 3.3).
4. Perform the first general inspection of the abdominal cavity (Fig. 3.4).

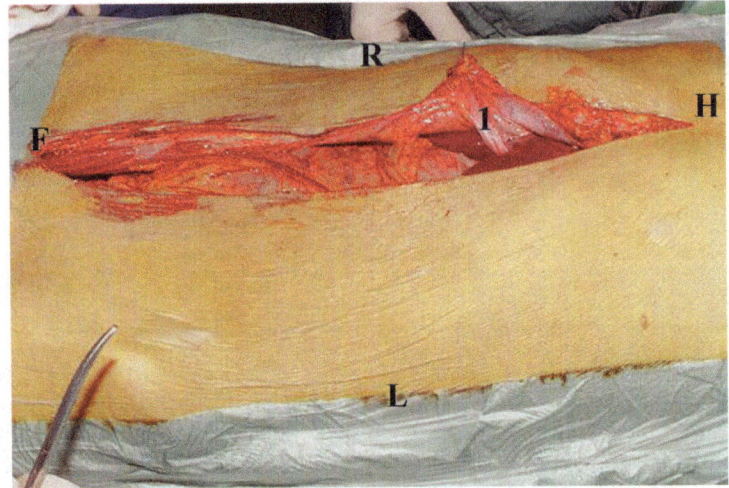

Fig. 3.1 Median laparotomy: 1 - Teres ligament, *H – head, F – feet, R – right, L – left*

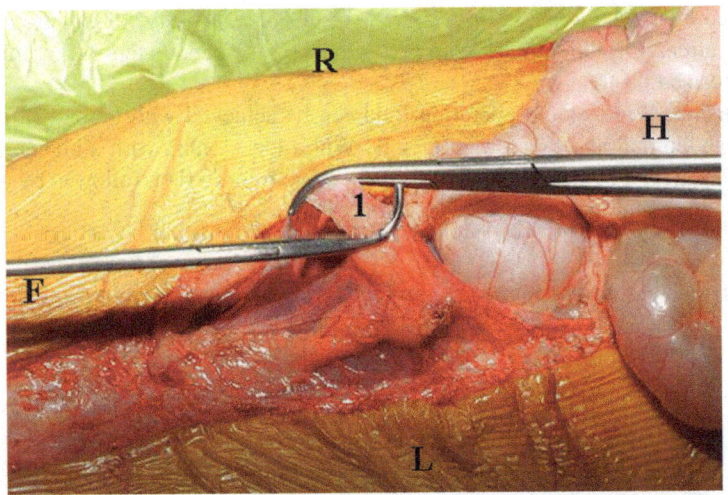

Fig. 3.2 1 - Teres ligament before cutting and ligation: *H – head, F – feet, R – right, L – left*

5. Free the diaphragm's tissues attached to the xiphoid process and the sternum (Fig. 3.5).
6. Reach with index finger the anterior mediastinum – retrosternal plane (behind xiphoid process and body of sternum) (Fig. 3.6a). If your finger is too short for developing the retrosternal plane, use a long blunt clamp (Fig. 3.6b).

3.1 Abdominal and Thoracic Incision

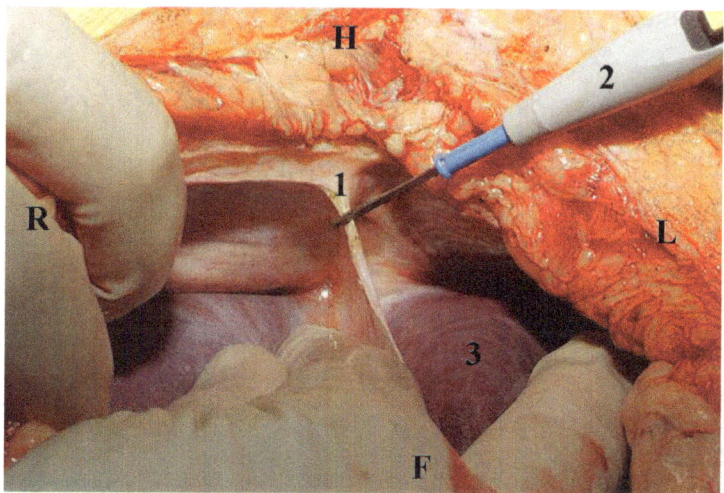

Fig. 3.3 1 - Falciform ligament: 2 – Electrocautery, 3 – Left liver lobe, *H – head, F – feet, R – right, L – left*

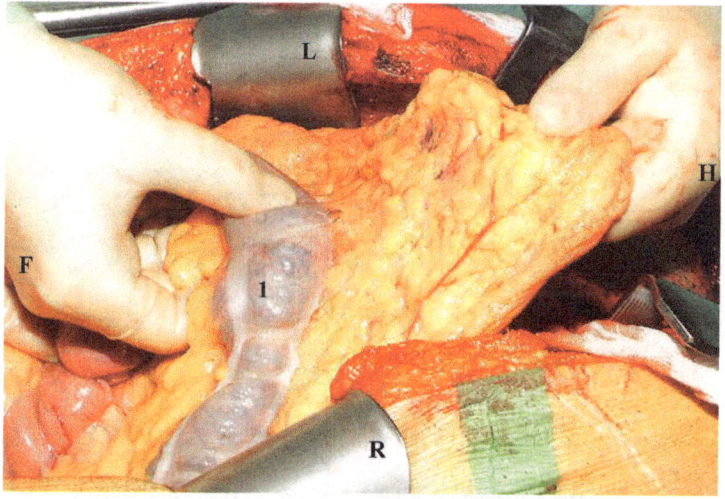

Fig. 3.4 First general abdominal inspection: 1 – Colon (elderly donors), *H – head, F – feet, R – right, L – left*

7. Always protect the liver with a large, wet, warm gauze (Fig. 3.7).

ATTENTION!
- Entering the abdomen through a previous laparotomy scars(s) can be difficult especially with an unstable donor; the safer incision would be beyond the old scar(s) where adhesions are less likely (1).

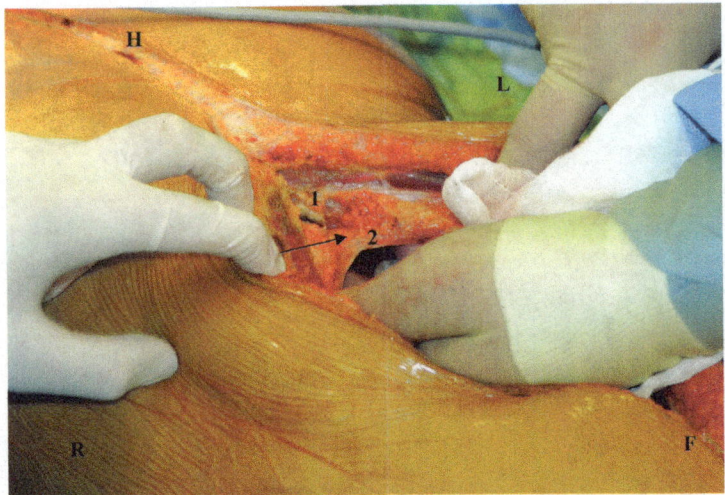

Fig. 3.5 Inferior part of sternotomy: 1 – xiphoid process, 2 – peritoneum, *H – head*, *R – right*, *F – feet*, *L –left*, – entrance to the anterior mediastinum (surface between the peritoneum and xiphoid process)

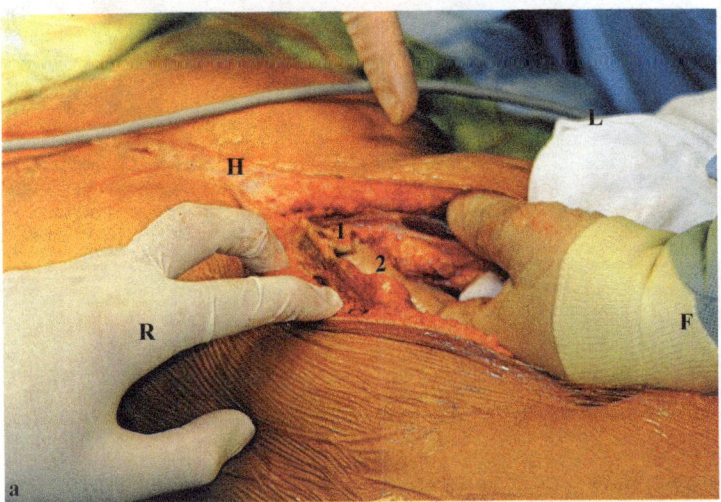

Fig. 3.6 a Inferior part of sternotomy: index finger behind the xiphoid process of the sternum: 1 – Xiphoid process, 2 – Index finger, *H – head*, *F – feet*, *R – right*, *L – left*

3.1 Abdominal and Thoracic Incision

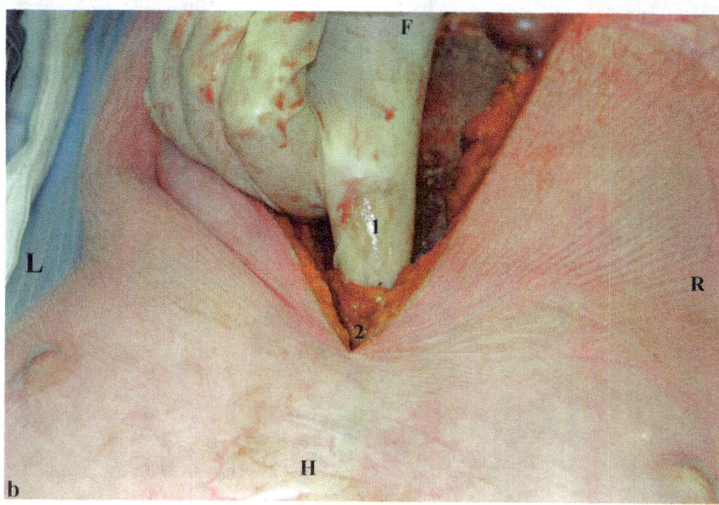

Fig. 3.6 (continued) **b** Inferior part of sternotomy: index finger extended anterior to the mediastinum: 1 – Finger index, 2 – Anterior mediastinum has been reached, *H – head, F – feet, R – right, L – left*

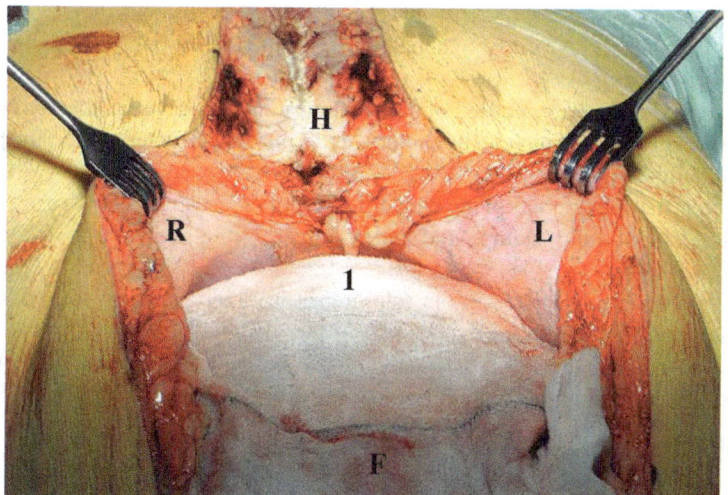

Fig. 3.7 Liver protected by a wet large gauze (1), *H – head, R – right, L – left, F – feet*

- Particularly with the older donors (above 65 years old) with a higher chance of abdominal malignancy, it could be useful to perform a median laparotomy first, followed by a general abdominal organ inspection (2).

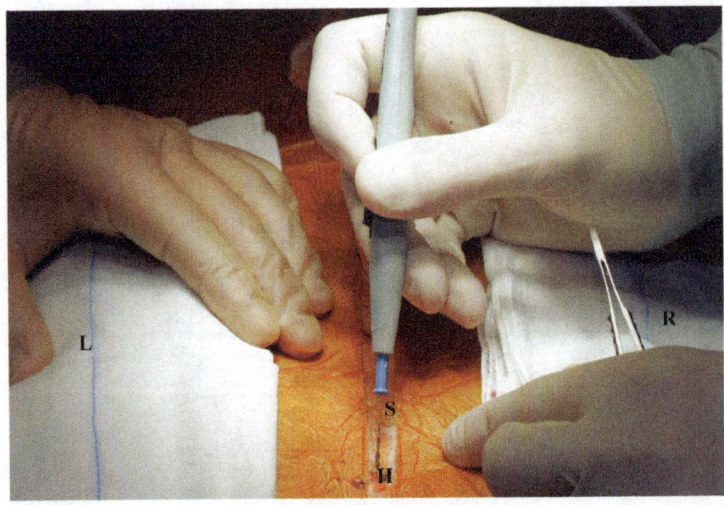

Fig. 3.8 Start median sternotomy, S – Sternum, H – head, L – left, R – right

3.1.2 Median Sternotomy

1. Start the incision 1–2 cm above manubrium sterni continuing up to the abdominal incision (Fig. 3.8).
2. Localise the superior border of the manubrium and develop the retrosternal plane from above using electrocautery, and your index finger – superior part of sternotomy (Fig. 3.9a, b).
3. Develop the retrosternal plane caudal to the xiphoid from below – use electrocautery, blunt long clamp, and index finger – inferior part of sternotomy (Fig. 3.10).
4. To cut the sternum, use scissors (children), pneumatic vertical sternal saw, or Gigli's saw (Fig. 3.11a, b).
5. Use sterile wax situated on the small gauze (application of friction) and electrocautery to obtain good sternum bone marrow hemostasis (Fig. 3.12a–c).

ATTENTION!
- To avoid liver, heart, lungs, and major vessel injury during sternotomy ask the anesthesiologist to lower the operating table and to stop ventilation
- During sternotomy avoid opening the pericardium and mediastinum pleura

3.1 Abdominal and Thoracic Incision

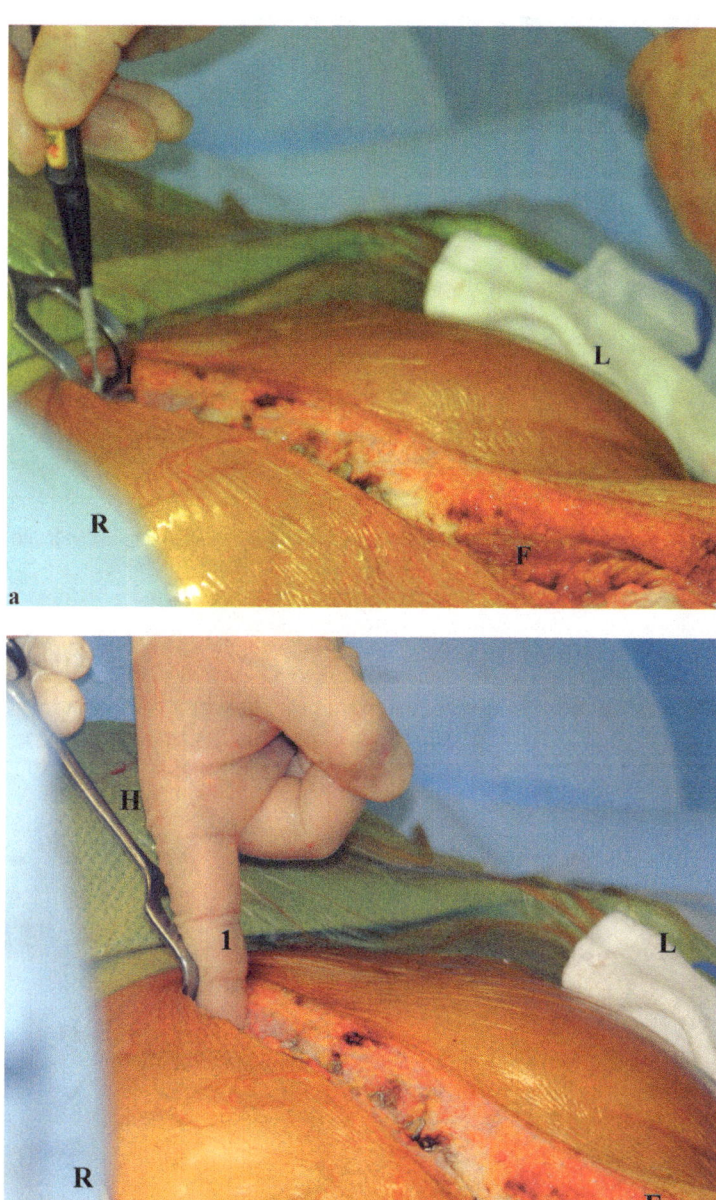

Fig. 3.9 a Superior part of sternotomy 1 – Superior border of the manubrium sterni, *L – left*, *R – right*, *F – feet*, **b** Superior part of sternotomy: developing the retrosternal plan with index finger behind the superior border of the manubrium sterni, *L – left*, *R – right*, *H – head*, *F – feet*

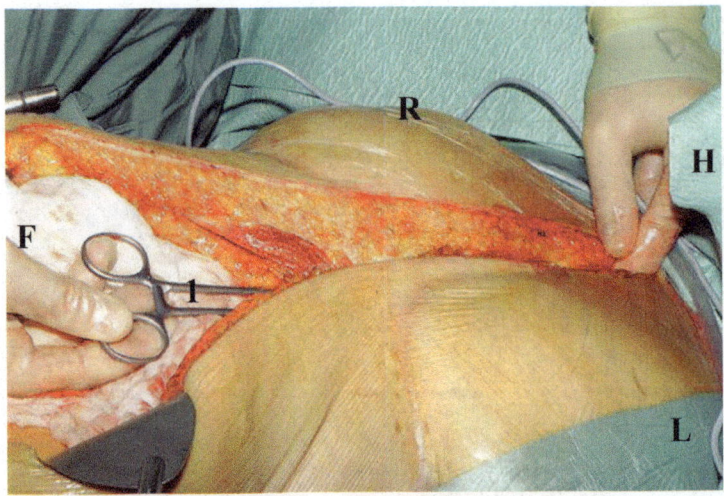

Fig. 3.10 Developing retrosternal space with the help of a long blunt clamp to catch and pull the Gigli's saw behind the sternum clamp: *L – left, R – right, H – head, F – feet*

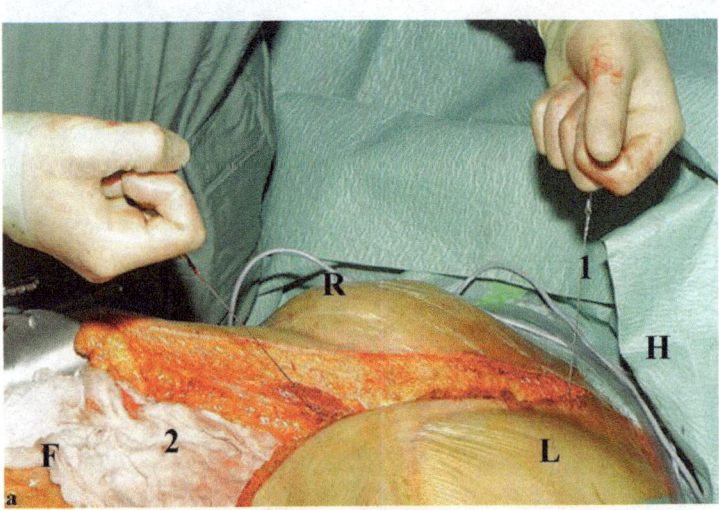

Fig. 3.11 a Sternotomy with the Gigli's saw: 1 – Gigli's saw, 2 – Protected liver, *H – head, F – feet, R – right, L – left*

3.1 Abdominal and Thoracic Incision

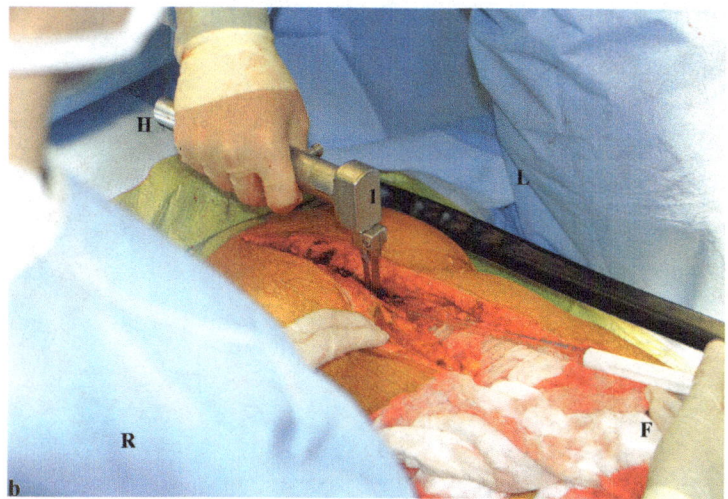

Fig. 3.11 (continued) **b** Sternotomy with pneumatic vertical saw: 1 – Pneumatic vertical saw, *H – head, F – feet, R – right, L – left*

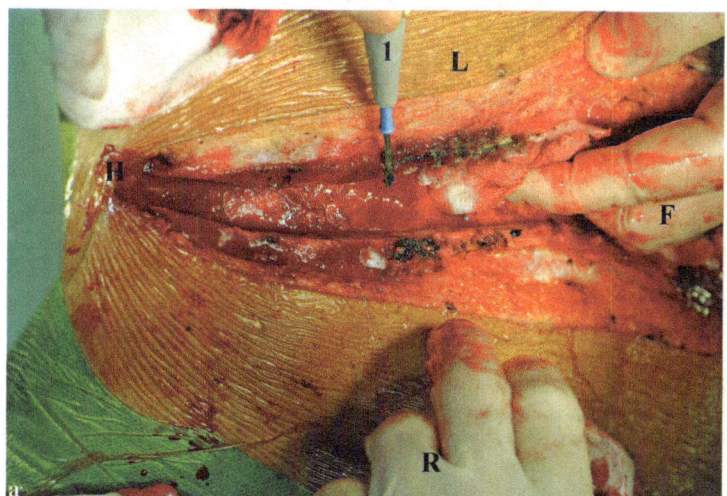

Fig. 3.12 a 1 – Electrocautery, 2 – Sternum, *H – head, F – feet, R – right, L – left*

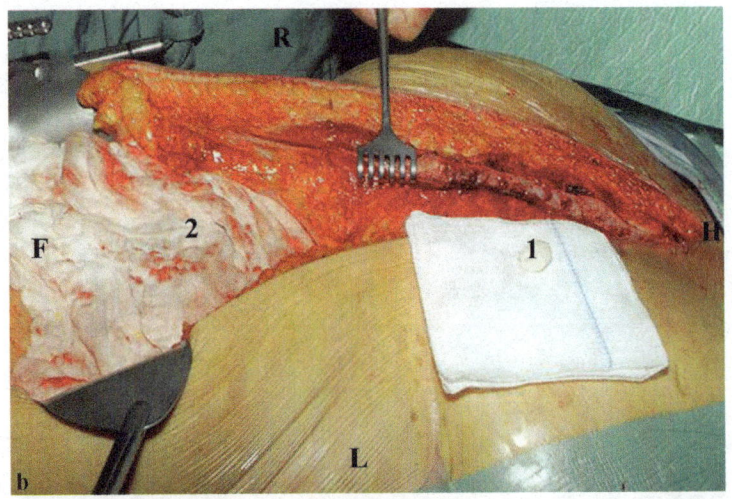

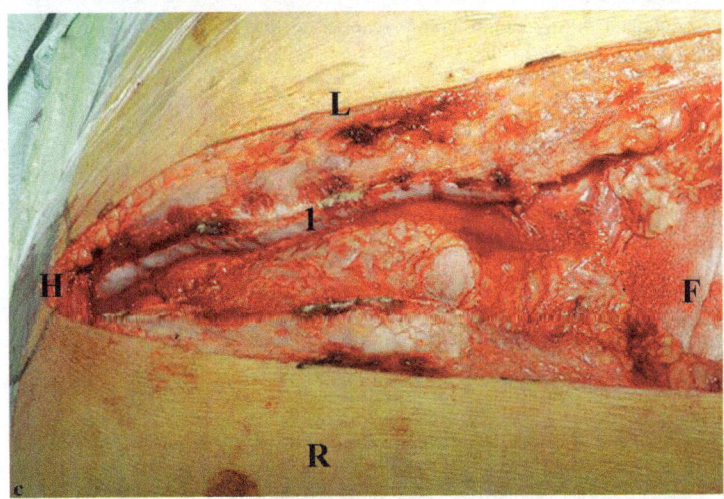

Fig. 3.12 (continued) **b** 1 – Sterile wax, 2 – Sterile wet gauze, *H – head, F – feet, R – right, L – left,* **c** Thanks to good hemostasis, there is no bleeding from the sternum: 1 – Sterile wax covers sternum surface, *H – head, F – feet, R – right, L – left*

3.1.3 Wide, Stable Thoracic and Abdomen Operating Field: The Retractors

1. With the thorax and abdominal retractor, slowly, gradually, try to obtain optimal exposure of the operating area (Fig. 3.13).
2. Cut on both sides of the diaphragm the sterno – costal part of the diaphragm up to the medioclavicular line (Fig. 3.14).

3.1 Abdominal and Thoracic Incision

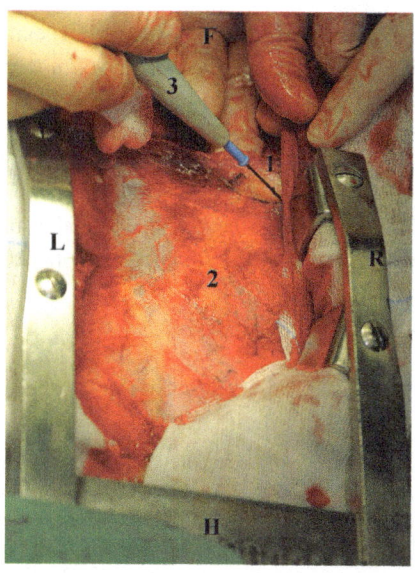

Fig. 3.13 1 – Sternocostal part of the diaphragma, 2 – Mediastinal pleura, 3 – Electrocautery, *H – head, F – feet, R – right, L – left*

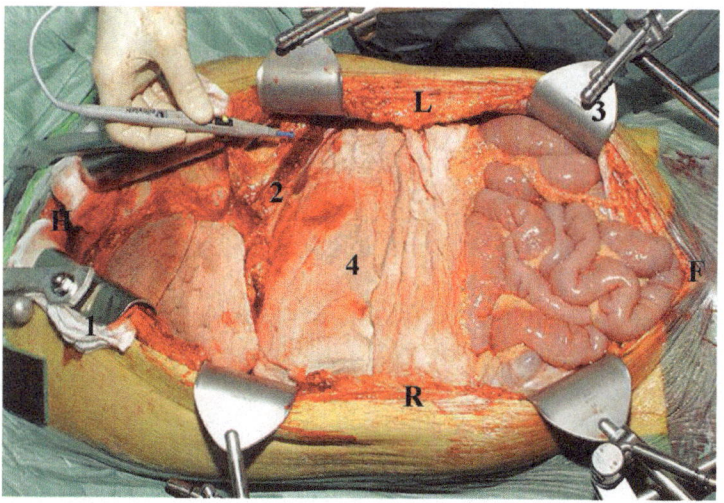

Fig. 3.14 1 – Thorax retractor, 2 – Sternocostal part of the diaphragm, 3 – Abdominal retractor, 4 – Liver always protected with a wet warm gauze, *H – head, F – feet, R – right, L – left*

ATTENTION!
- With a very small thorax retractor opening in steps, visualization of the anterior mediastinum must be carried out very carefully to obtain optimal exposure while avoiding fractures of sternum and ribs.
- Opening of the pericardium and mediastinal pleura with the retractors should be avoided during the creation of a wide operating field for abdominal organ dissection.
- If lung inspection is necessary (in case of questionable thoracic organ quality) the mediastinal pleura and pericardial sack may be opened.

Literature

1. Hirshberg A, Mattox KL (2005) The crash laparotomy. In the Top Knife the Art & Craft of Trauma Surgery, TFM Publishing, Castle Hill Barns, Harley, 53–70
2. Buell JF, Alloway RR, Woodle ES (2006) How can donors with previous malignancy be evaluated? Forum on Liver Transplantation. Journal of Hepatology 45:483–513

Chapter 4
Detailed and Thorough Abdominal Organ Inspection

Abstract Background: Generally, inspection of abdominal organs should include liver, pancreas, stomach, small bowel, colon, and pelvis. In women, attention should be paid to the pelvis with careful inspection of the ovaries and uterus. During organ inspection, attention should be also given to the enlarged lymph nodes in the iliac fossa, small bowel mesentery, para-aortic region, hepatoduodenal ligament, and liver hilus. Each organ should be carefully inspected. The final decision about which organs can be accepted for transplantation has to be taken by the procurement surgeon. In difficult cases, additional medical investigation and communication with the recipient centre will help the procurement surgeon make the right decision.

Conclusion: An organ transplanted with a primary cancer or cancer metastases causes not only a great dilemma for the recipient, but also for the recipient team to retransplant or observe. To avoid such a situation, detailed and thorough organ inspection both during and after organ procurement is in every case, strongly recommended.

Keywords Organ inspection, Abdomen inspection, Organ procurement, Liver inspection, Pancreas inspection, Steatosis, Oedema, Blood supply, Examination blood supply, Gut inspection

4.1 Introduction

Generally, inspection of the abdominal cavity should include liver, pancreas, stomach, small bowel, colon, and pelvis. In women, special attention should be paid to the pelvis with careful inspection of the ovaries and uterus. During abdominal organ inspection, attention should be also given to the enlarged lymph nodes in the iliac fossa, small bowel mesentery, para-aortic region, hepatoduodenal ligament, and liver hilum. An occasional dilemma faced by organ procurement teams is the discovery of an incidental renal cell carcinoma after the removal of the organ.

These lesions are often discovered during back-table or accidentally after transplantation.

An organ transplanted from a donor with cancer is not only a great dilemma for the recipient but also for the recipient team – whether to retransplant or how to follow-up. To avoid such a situation, detailed and thorough organ inspection during and after organ procurement is strongly indicated (1, 2, 3, 4).

4.2 Liver

4.2.1 General Examination

1. Contour
2. Colour
3. Consistency

4.2.2 Size of the Liver (Fig. 4.1)

1. Size of the donor and the recipient must be taken into account.
2. Size is a particular concern in split and pediatric liver transplantation.

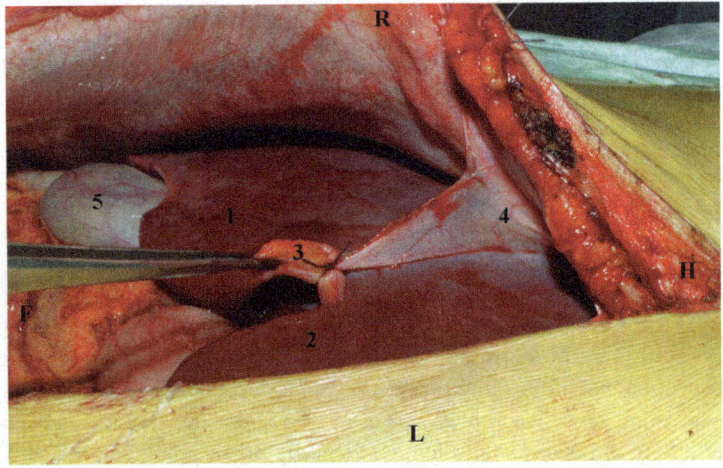

Fig. 4.1 Normal liver. 1 – Right liver lobe, 2 – Left liver lobe, 3 – Teres ligament, 4 – Falciform ligament, 5 – Gallbladder, *H – head, F – feet, R – right, L – left*

4.2 Liver

4.2.3 *Parenchyma Inspection with Respect to Micro and Macrosteatosis*

1. Micro – or macrosteatosis, which is worse?

ATTENTION!
- Liver steatosis is strongly associated, after transplantation, with poor graft function. Mild to moderate steatosis does not reduce the success rate of liver transplantation and is similar to those achieved with normal function. Livers with more than 40–50% macrosteatosis should not be used. Macrovesical steatosis is often the result of acute injury and could be reversible, but more than 15% results in impaired post-transplant function (1, 2, 3).
- Microvesicular steatosis seems to have a low impact on the postoperative liver function. Consequent to such findings, liver biopsy should be performed, but in small hospitals, a pathologist is frequently not available during the night. The best option is to communicate with the recipient centre where, in most of the cases, a pathologist is available during the night (1–4). Finally, in all such cases, the procurement surgeon has to make the definitive decision. A percutaneous liver biopsy performed at the bedside, before organ procurement may help prevent unnecessary donor laparotomy (3, 4).

3. Cirrhosis – if not evident, you need the assistance of a pathologist to be able to take the final decision. Contact the local pathologist or recipient centre.
4. Fibrosis – here too, you need a pathologist's input before you can make the final decision. Contact recipient centre.
5. Edema (hypernatremia, hypoalbuminemia, high central venous pressure, and injury). In my experience of organ donation, definitive decision making is possible only after cold organ perfusion.
6. Injury (tear, hematoma, bleeding, and biliary leak) – final decision can be taken before or after cold organ perfusion.
7. Tumor (benign, malignant) – you need a pathologist's report before taking the final decision. Contact recipient center.
8. Infections (cholecystitis, cholangitis, hepatitis) – a bacteriologist can give you a quick analysis of the infection.

ATTENTION!
- Main adhesions to the liver capsule and/or to the gallbladder have to be gently freed during initial organ inspection (to avoid damage during liver procurement).
- Swollen liver during organ retrieval because of high central venous pressure – in my experience in such a case, a combination of 20% albumin and lasix (furosemide) may be helpful.
- Still swollen liver after albumin and lasix treatment – delay any final decision until after cold organ perfusion. In most of the cases the liver will change shape, consistency and become smaller with a wedge shape.

- Remember that after good VCI decompression and cold organ perfusion, only high steatotic and fibrotic liver will not change the shape, colour, and consistency.

4.2.4 Examination of Arterial Blood Supply to the Liver

1. Perform a careful examination of the hepatogastric (Fig. 4.2) and hepatoduodenal ligament (Fig. 4.3).

ATTENTION!
There is confusion in the anatomical and surgical literature regarding the following terms: aberrant, replacing and accessory artery. The distinction can be explained in a simple way: an aberrant artery could be accessory or replacing but not inversely (7, 8, 9, 10, 11, 12, 13, 14).

Van Damme does not follow Michel's (14) distinction; according to him, during surgery, it is very difficult to distinguish between a replaced or accessory artery. He uses only one term concerning anatomic variations of hepatic artery – the aberrant artery (7, 8, 9).

According to the following literature (7, 8, 9, 10, 11, 12, 13, 14), and taking into account the anatomical frequency of occurrence of the normal and aberrant hepatic arteries, I have made my own classification which I hope might be helpful during organ procurement:

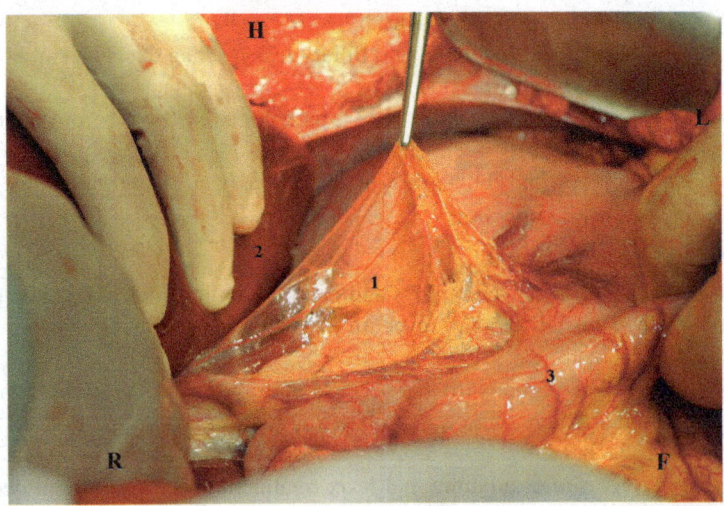

Fig. 4.2 1 – Hepatogastric ligament, 2 – Left liver lobe, 3 – Stomach, *H – head, F – feet, R – right, L – left*

4.2 Liver

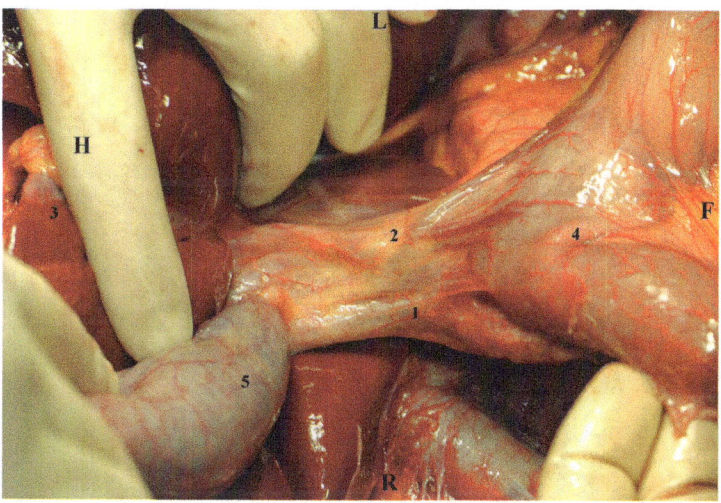

Fig. 4.3 Hepatoduodenal ligament. 1 – Common bile duct, 2 – Region of the hepatic artery, 3 – Liver, 4 – Duodenum, 5 – Gallbladder, *H – head, F – feet, R – right, L – left*

- *First* – a normal liver arterial blood supply (NLABS) means that celiac trunk is coming from the abdominal aorta, common hepatic artery is coming from the celiac trunk, proper hepatic artery is coming from the common hepatic artery and there are no additional arterial branches supporting liver (Fig. 4.4).
- *Second* – the left aberrant hepatic artery is coming from the left gastric artery, celiac trunk and there is the NLABS (Fig. 4.5).
- *Third* – the right aberrant hepatic artery is coming from the superior mesenteric artery (SMA) and there is the NLABS (Fig. 4.6).
- *Fourth* – patient has both right and left aberrant hepatic arteries and there is the NLABS (Fig. 4.7).
- There are also a lot of other anomalies of the liver arterial blood supply, such as, for example, an entire common (replaced) hepatic artery coming from the SMA; in this case, there is no celiac trunk and no common hepatic artery.
- During inspection, use your fingers for palpation and your mind to *see* and feel three dimensionally the anatomical structures with their consistency, form, pulsation, and position in relation to the other structures and organs in the abdominal cavity.
- The arterial blood supply of the liver can sometimes surprise not only the procurement surgeon, but also an experienced transplant surgeon.
- If you want to be good, prepare yourself for all anatomic variations. To help you, please read the following literature (7, 8, 9, 10, 11).

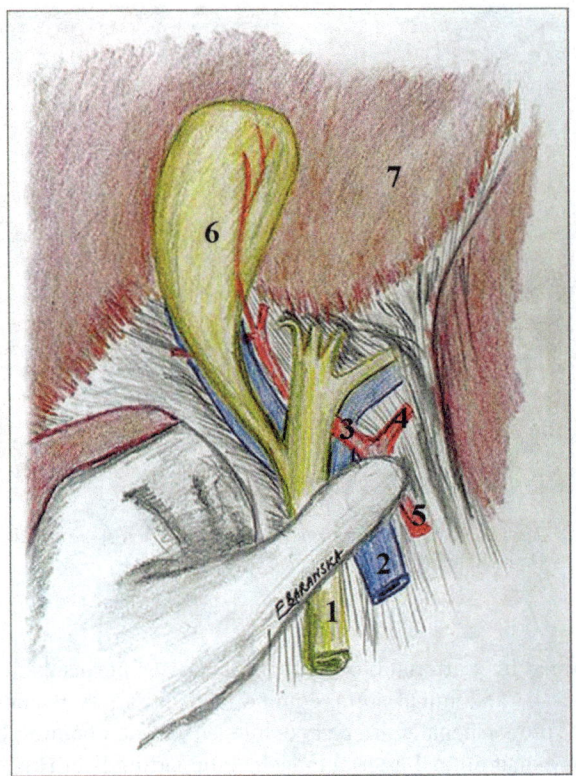

Fig. 4.4 Hepatoduodenal ligament. 1 – Liver normal arterial blood supply common bile duct, 2 – Portal vein, 3 – Proper hepatic artery, 4 – Common hepatic artery, 5 – Gastroduodenal artery, 6 – Gallbladder, 7 – Liver

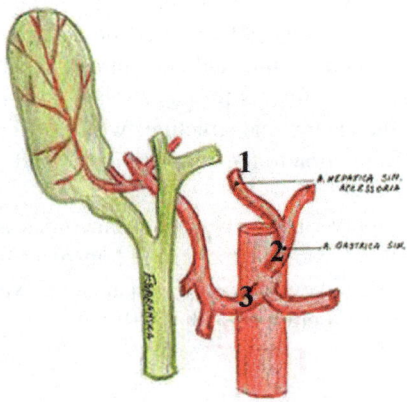

Fig. 4.5 1 – Left aberrant hepatic artery, 2 – Left gastric artery, 3 – Common hepatic artery

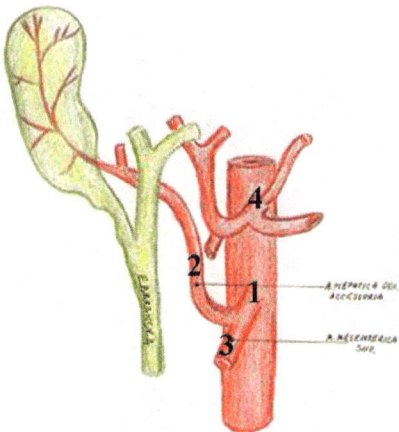

Fig. 4.6 1 and 3 – Superior mesenteric artery, 2 – Right aberrant hepatic artery, 4 – Celiac trunk

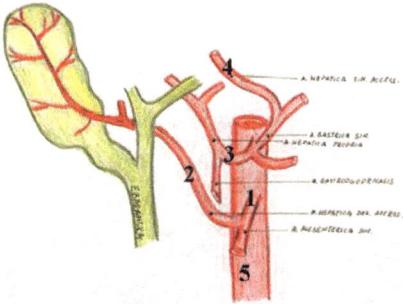

Fig. 4.7 1 – Superior mesenteric artery, 2 – Right aberrant hepatic artery, 3 – Common hepatic artery, 4 – Left aberrant hepatic artery, 5 – Abdominal aorta

4.3 The Pancreas

4.3.1 Routes for Surgical Access

1. Through the hepatogastric ligament – remember that here the left accessory or the replaced hepatic artery might be found (Fig. 4.8).
2. Through gastrocolic ligament – to be found attached between the greater curvature of the stomach spleen and transverse colon. In the left side of the abdomen in the region of stomach, spleen, transverse colon is almost transparent and there are almost no vessels. This is a good place to make an opening with electrocautery and access the left side of the pancreas for inspection (Fig. 4.9a, b).

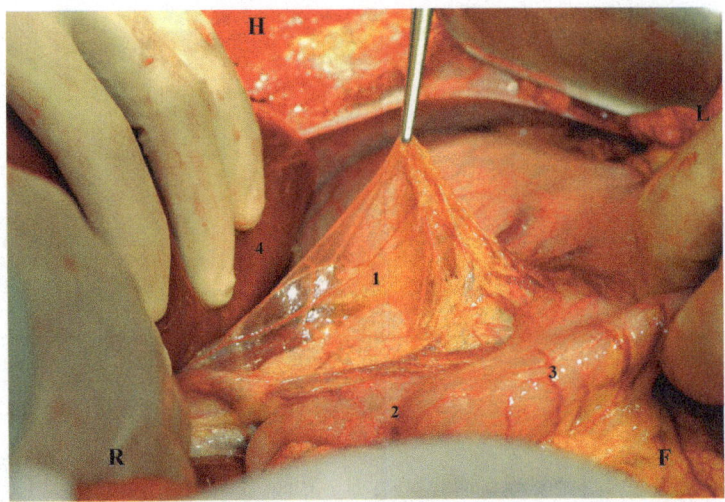

Fig. 4.8 1 – Hepatogastric ligament, 2 – Pylorus, 3 – Stomach, 4 – Liver, *H – head, F – feet, R – right, L – left*

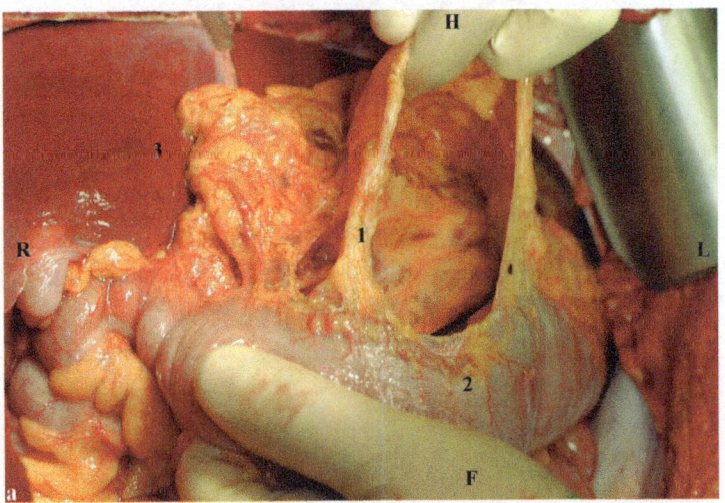

Fig. 4.9 a 1 – Gastrocolic ligament, 2 – Transverse colon, 3 – Liver, *H – head, F – feet, R – right, L – left*

4.3 The Pancreas

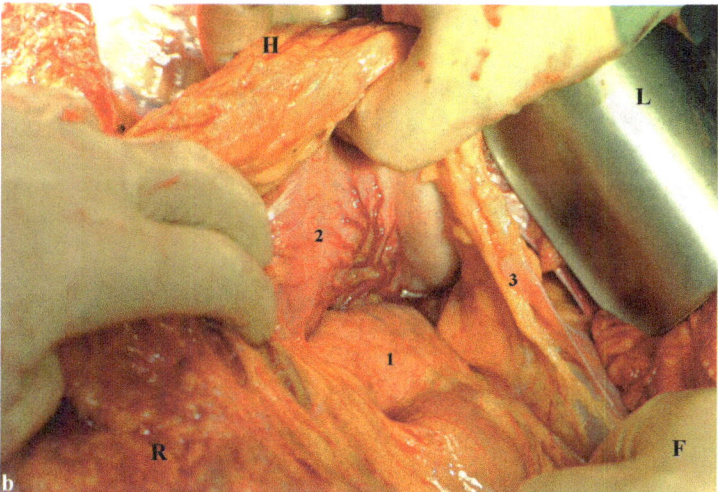

Fig. 4.9 (continued) **b** 1 – Pancreas, 2 – Stomach posterior wall, 3 – Gastrocolic ligament, *H – head, F – feet, R – right, L – left*

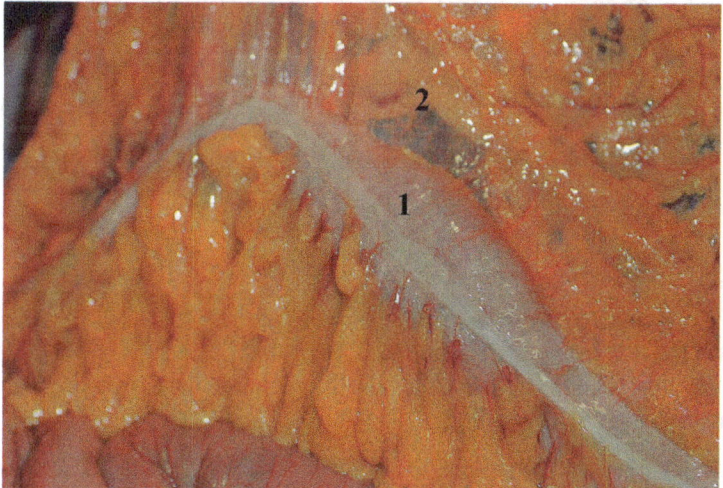

Fig. 4.10 Detaching the greater omentum. 1 – Posterior side of the transverse colon, 2 – Greater omentum

3. By detaching the greater omentum from the transverse colon (Fig. 4.10) in some cases, for example, in obese donors and also for donors who have had abdominal operations can be very difficult.
4. By extended Kocher manoeuver (Fig. 4.11). The peritoneum is incised in the lateral side of the duodenum, and the duodenum with the pancreas head could be pulled up and placed to the left side of the abdomen (for details see Chap. 5).

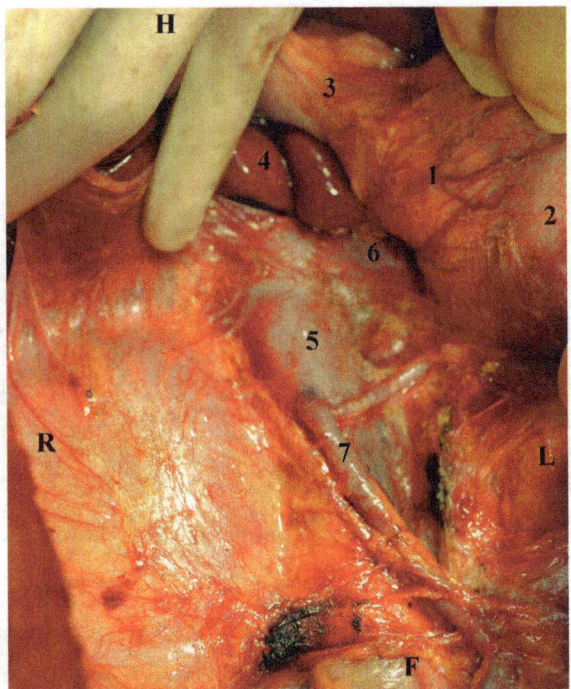

Fig. 4.11 Extended Kocher manoeuvre. 1 – Posterior side of the pancreas head, 2 – Duodenum, 3 – Hepatoduodenal ligament, 4 – Liver, 5 – IVC, 6 – Left renal vein, 7 – Gonadal vein, *H – head, F – feet, R – right, L – left* (for more details see Chap. 5)

ATTENTION!
During organ procurement, in every case, always choose the easiest surgical access for pancreas inspection.

4.3.2 Pancreas Inspection – Organ Assessment

1. Colour – normal light tan or pinkish
2. Anatomic variations of the right aberrant hepatic artery (14, 15)
3. Interlobular oedema
4. Consistency
5. Tumour(s)
6. Mechanical injury of the pancreatic parenchyma and/or the spleen
7. Infection and inflammation

ATTENTION!
- During pancreas inspection use *no touch* technique.
- If necessary, gently and delicately, palpate.

4.4 Inspection of Other Abdominal Organs

4.4.1 Gut Inspection

1. Inspect the rest of the abdominal organs from the oesophagus until the rectum.
2. In donors above 50 years, give special attention to the pelvis and large bow, paying attention to possible malignancy and/or infection.

4.4.2 Additional Investigations During Organ Inspection

1. Needle or open biopsy (Fig. 4.12)
2. Quick pathological examination (frozen section in the donor or recipient hospital)
3. Intraoperative or back table ultrasonography (liver, pancreas, kidney)
4. Bacteriological examination

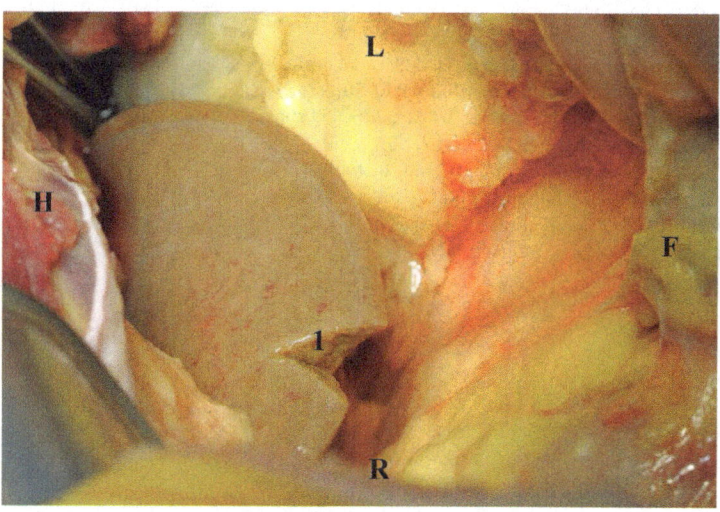

Fig. 4.12 Liver steatosis open biopsy was made. 1 – Biopsied tissue, *H – head, F – feet, R – right, L – left*

Literature

1. Buell JF, Alloway RR, Woodle ES (2006) How can donors with previous malignancy be evaluated? Forum on Liver Transplantation. Journal of Hepatology: 45: 483-513
2. Urena MA, Ruiz-Delgado FC, Gonzalez EM et al (1998) Assessing risk of the use of livers with macro and microsteatosis in a liver transplant program. Transplant Proceeding: 30: 7: 3288-3291
3. D'Alessandro AM, Kalayoglu M, Sollinger HW et al (1991) The predictive value of donor liver biopsies on the development of primary nonfunction after orthotopic liver transplantation. Transplant Proceeding: 23: 1536-1537
4. Urena MA, Moreno Gonzalez E, Romero CJ et al (1999) An approach to the rational use of steatotic donor livers in liver transplantation. Hepatogastroenterology: 46(26): 1164-1173.
5. Fernandez ED, Schmidt M, Bittinger F, Mauer D (2007) Intraoperative assessment of liver organ condition by the procurement surgeon. Transplantation Proceedings: 39: 1485-1487
6. Fishbein TM, Fiel MI, Emre S et al (1997) Use of livers with microvesicular fat safely expands the donor pool. Transplantation: 64(2): 248-251
7. Skandalakis JE, Branum GD, Colborn GL, Weidman TA, Skandalakis PN, Skandalakis LJ, Zoras O (2004) Extrahepatic biliary tract and gallbladder. In Skandalakis JE, Weidman TA, Foster RS Jr, Kingsnorth AN, Skandalakis LJ, Skandalakis PN, Mirilas PS (eds) Skandalakis' Surgical Anatomy. The Embryologic and Anatomic Basis of Modern Surgery, Vol. II, Paschalidis Medical Publications, Athens, pp 1093-1150
8. Van Damme JP, Bonte J (eds) (1990) Part one: the celiac trunk and its branches. Vascular Anatomy in Abdominal Surgery, Thieme Medical Publisher, New York, pp 4-47
9. Nghiem DD (1989) A technique for concomitant whole duodeno-pancreatectomy and hepatectomy for transplantation in the multiple organ donor. Surgery Gynecology and Obstetrics: 169: 257-258
10. Van Damme JP, Bonte J (1985) The branches of the celiac trunk, Acta Anatomica: 122: 104-115
11. Skandalakis JE, Branum GD, Colborn GL, Mirilas PS, Weidman TA, Skandalakis LJ, Kingsnorth AN, Zora O (2004) Liver. In Skandalakis PN, Weidman TA, Foster RS Jr, Kingsnorth AN, Skandalakis LJ, Skandalakis PN, Mirilas PS (eds) Skandalakis' Surgical Anatomy. The Embryologic and Anatomic Basis of Modern Surgery, vol. II, Paschalidis Medical Publications, Athens, pp 1005-1092
12. Suzuki T, Nakayasu A, Kawabe K et al (1971) Surgical significance of anatomic variations of the hepatic artery. The American Journal of Surgery: 122: 505-512
13. Sakorafas GH, Friess H, Balsiger BM et al (2001) Problems of reconstruction during pancreatoduodenectomy. Digestive Surgery: 18: 363-369
14. Michels NA (1955) Blood supply and anatomy of the upper abdominal organs with the descriptive atlas, J.B.Lippincott, Philadelphia, PA
15. Furukawa H, Shimada K, Iwata R, et al (2000) A replaced common hepatic artery through the pancreatic parenchyma. Surgery: 127: 711-712

Chapter 5
Retroperitoneal Right-Sided Visceral Mobilisation: The Cattel–Braasch Manoeuvre

Abstract Background: The Cattel–Braasch manoeuvre is based on the anatomical observation that the small mesentery is attached to the posterior abdominal wall along a short oblique line of fusion. The Cattel–Braasch manoeuvre begins at the common bile duct and ends at the ligament of Treitz. It allows you to mobilise the whole duodenum, pancreas head, small bowel and the right colon and bring the two last structures outside the abdomen. Thanks to anatomical knowledge of the avascular planes – the Cattel–Braasch manoeuvre is the one of the quickest mobilisation surgical techniques with minimal blood loss. Extended Kocher's manoeuvre is a part of Cattel–Braasch manoeuvre and generally consists of full exposition of the inferior vena cava (IVC), renal veins, abdominal aorta, and superior mesenteric artery (SMA).

Conclusion: The Cattel–Braasch manoeuvre, when completed, can allow very good access to the entire retroperinoneum with access to the following organs and structures: abdominal aorta below the SMA, IVC, SMA, inferior mesenteric artery (IMA), inferior mesenteric vein (IMV), whole duodenum, pancreas head, left adrenal gland and the left adrenal vein, celiac plexus, both kidneys, ureters and common and external iliac vessels.

Keywords Cattel–Braasch manoeuvre, Kocher manoeuvre, Right-sided visceral rotation, Colon and small bowel mobilisation, Pancreas head mobilisation

5.1 Introduction

The Cattel–Braasch manoeuvre is based on the anatomical observation that the small mesentery is attached to the posterior abdominal wall along a short oblique line of fusion called the *white line* of Toldt (1). The white line of Toldt consists of peritoneal reflection at the area of the lateral wall of the cecum and ascending colon (2). The Cattel–Braasch manoeuvre begins at the common bile duct and ends at the ligament of Treitz. It allows very good mobilisation of whole duodenum and pancreas head, the small and the large bowel and to place the last two of them outside the abdomen (1,2,3).

Extended Kocher's manoeuvre, which is a part of Cattel–Braasch manoeuvre and generally consists of total duodenum and pancreas head mobilisation, gives full exposition of the right kidney with hilum, renal veins, IVC abdominal aorta, celiak plexus, and superior mesenteric artery (SMA).

5.2 Right Colon Mobilisation

5.2.1 Surgical Steps

1. Ask the assistant to lift up and gently pull the ascending colon to the left side of the abdomen (Fig.5.1).
2. Use the electrocautery and cut the lateral parietal peritoneum from the right iliac external artery up to the hepatoduodenal ligament (Fig. 5.2a, b).
3. If necessary, localise and mark the right ureter with the vessel loop; the right ureter and the gonadal vessels have to be separated from the mesocolic plane (Fig. 5.2b).

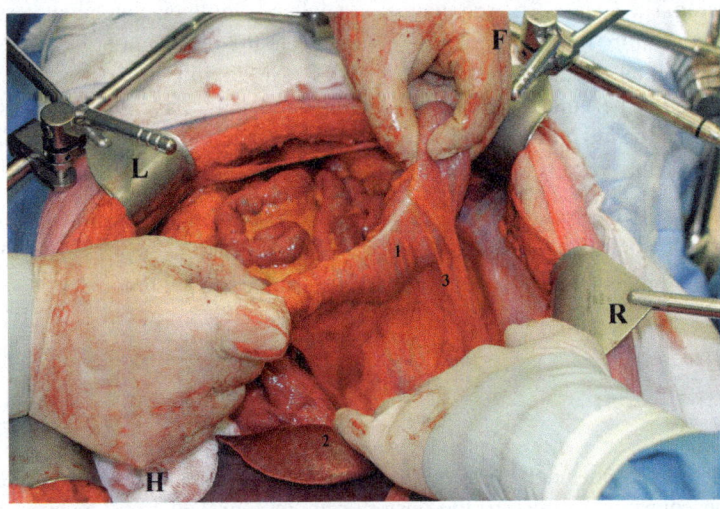

Fig. 5.1 1 – Ascending colon, 2 – Liver, 3 – Peritoneum, *H – head, F – feet, R – right, L – left*

5.2 Right Colon Mobilisation

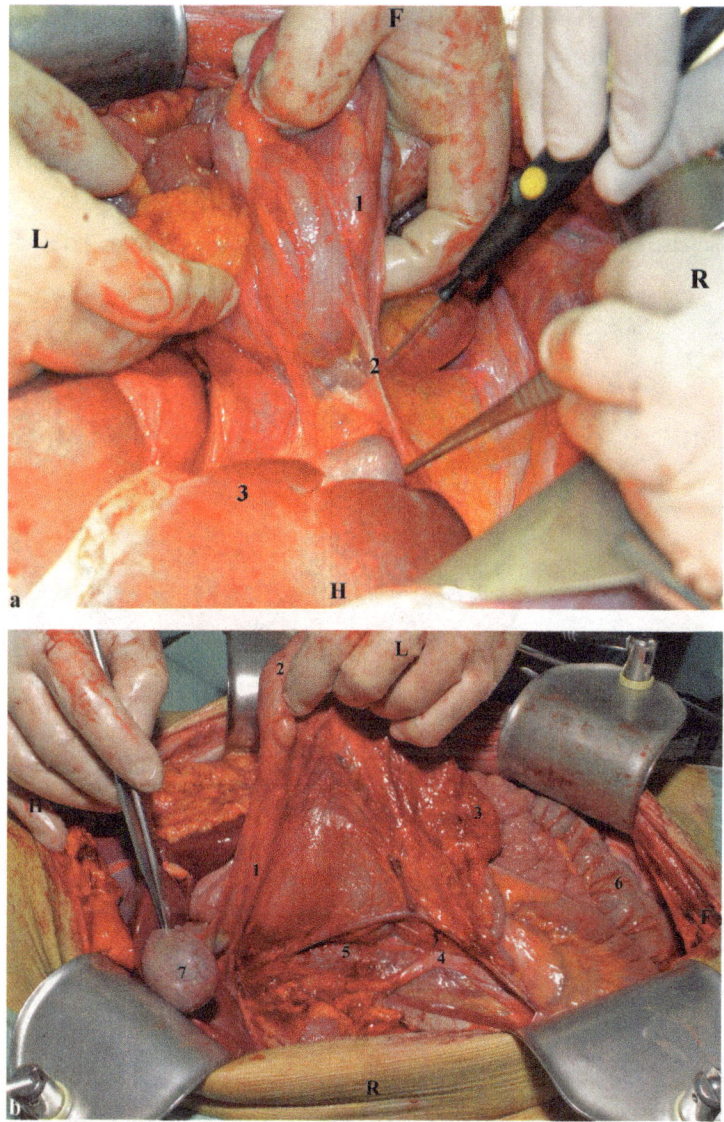

Fig. 5.2 a 1 – Ascending colon, 2 – Peritoneum with line of Toldt, 3 – Liver, *H – head, F – feet, R – right, L – left,* **b** 1 – Transverse colon, 2 – Ascending colon, 3 – Cecum, 4 – Ureter, 5 – IVC, 6 – Sigmoid, 7 – Gallbladder, *H – head, F – feet, R – right, L – left*

5.3 Extended Kocher Manoeuvre – Duodenopancreatic Mobilisation

5.3.1 Surgical Steps

1. Cut the peritoneum at the right side of the duodenum (Fig. 5.3).
2. Cut the inferior avascular border of the foramen omentale (Winslow) (Fig. 5.4).

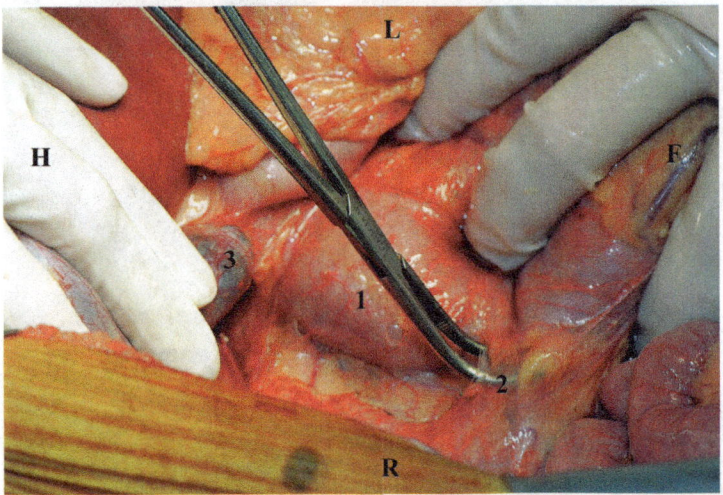

Fig. 5.3 1 – Duodenum, 2 – Peritoneum on the right side of the duodenum, 3 – Gallbladder, *H – head, F – feet, R – right, L – left*

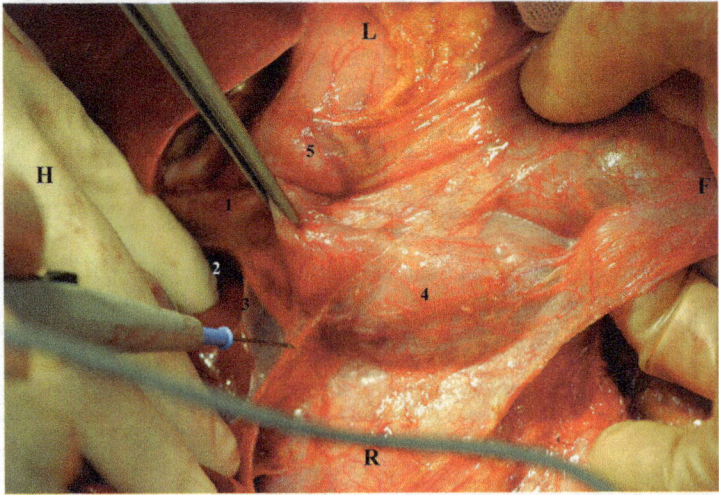

Fig. 5.4 1 – Hepatoduodenal ligament, 2 – Foramen ovale (Winslow), 3 – Inferior avascular border of the foramen ovale, 4 – Duodenum, 5 – Stomach, *H – head, F – feet, R – right, L – left*

5.3 Extended Kocher Manoeuvre – Duodenopancreatic Mobilisation 49

3. Cut the avascular surface between inferior vena cava (IVC) and the posterior side of the pancreas head and the duodenum and mobilise them up to the SMA and abdominal aorta (Fig. 5.5, 5.6, 5.7).

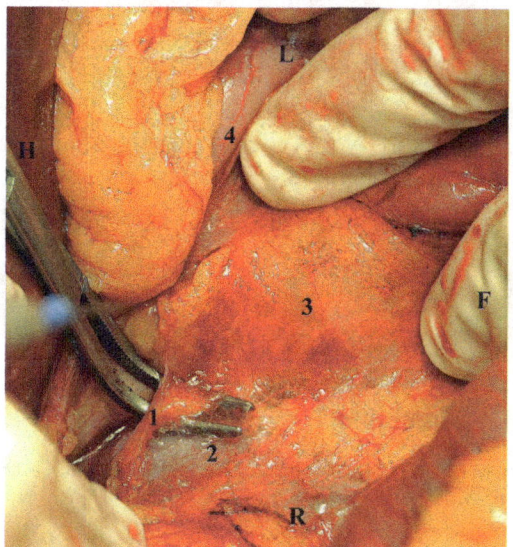

Fig. 5.5 1 – The rest of avascular inferior border of the foramen ovale, 2 – IVC, 3 – Posterior side of the pancreas head, 4 – Duodenums, *H – head, F – feet, R – right, L – left*

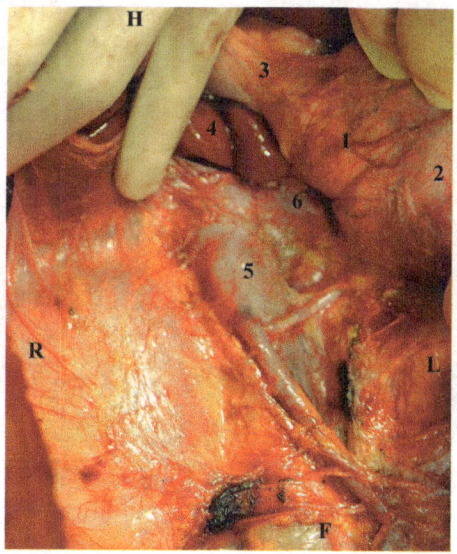

Fig. 5.6 1 – Posterior side of the pancreas head, 2 – Duodenum posterior side, 3 – Hepatoduodenal ligament, 4 – Liver, 5 – IVC, 6 – Left renal vein, *H – head, F – feet, R – right, L – left*

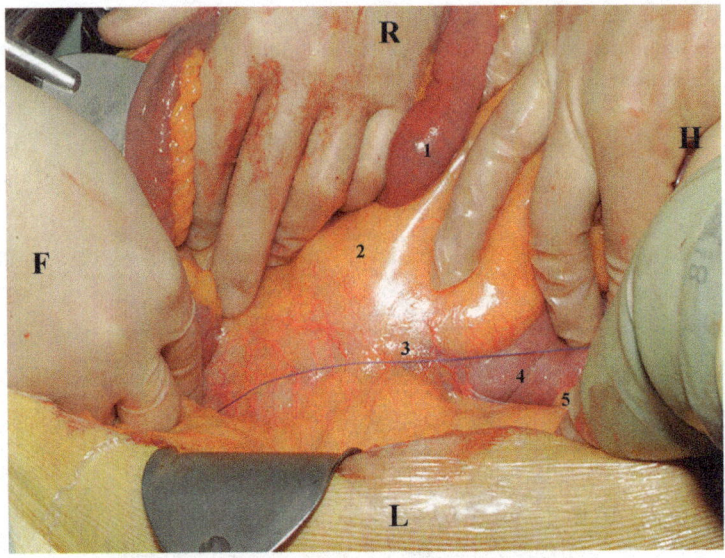

Fig. 5.7 1 – Small bowel, 2 – Small bowel mesentery, 3 – Peritoneum, 4 – Duodenum, 5 – Treitz ligament, *H – head, F – feet, R – right, L – left*

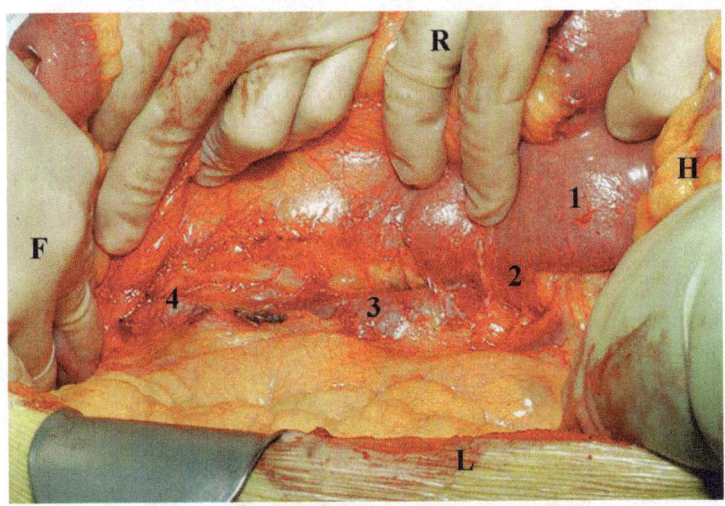

Fig. 5.8 1 – Duodenum, 2 – The rest of the Treitz ligament, 3 – IVC, 4 – Right common iliac artery, *H – head, F – feet, R – right, L – left*

5.4 Small Bowel Mobilisation

5.4.1 Surgical Steps

1. Place the mobilised right colon, duodenum and the head of the pancreas in the physiological position, back to the right side of the abdomen.
2. Move the small bowel to the right side of the abdomen.
3. Visualise parietal peritoneum between the Treitz ligament and right iliac external artery (Fig. 5.7).
4. Cut the peritoneum starting from the ligament of Treitz up to the distal part of the right iliac external artery (Fig. 5.8).
5. From the right iliac vessels up to the SMA free the small bowel completely from the retroperinoneum.
6. Place mobilised colon and small bowel on the upper abdomen and the thorax, cover the bowels with wet gauze (Fig. 5.9) to fix them, use the blades of the abdominal retractor or ask the assistant to hold them (Fig. 5.10).

ATTENTION!
- Avoid torsion of the colon and the small bowel mesentery as this may cause ischemia to them.
- Pay close attention to the blood perfusion of the small bowel and the colon.

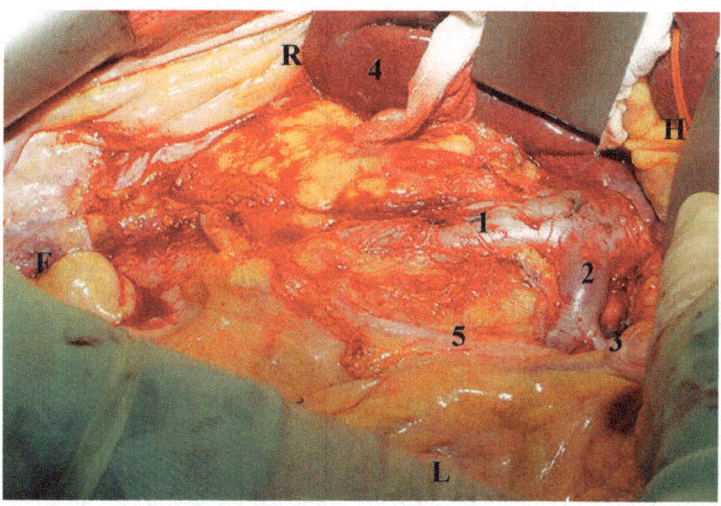

Fig. 5.9 1 – IVC, 2 – Left renal vein, 3 – Left adrenal vein, 4 – Liver, 5 – Inferior mesenteric vein(IMV), *H – head, F – feet, R – right, L – left*

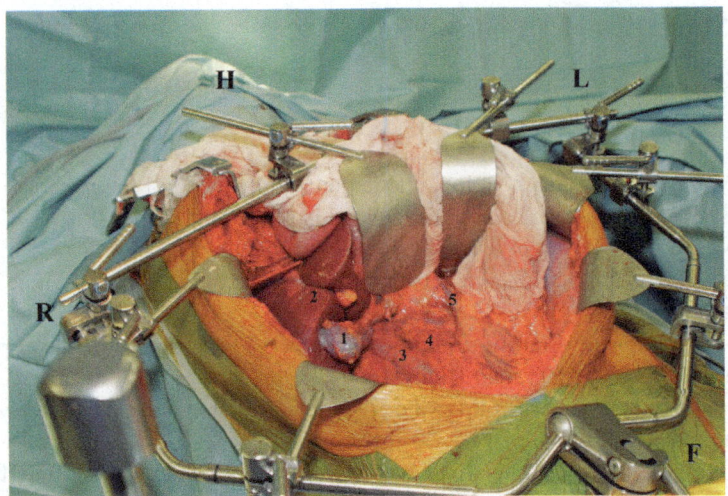

Fig. 5.10 To fix the small bowel and the colon, retractor blades were used. 1 – Gallbladder, 2 – Liver, 3 – IVC, 4 – Aorta, 5 – IMV, *H – head, F – feet, R – right, L – left*

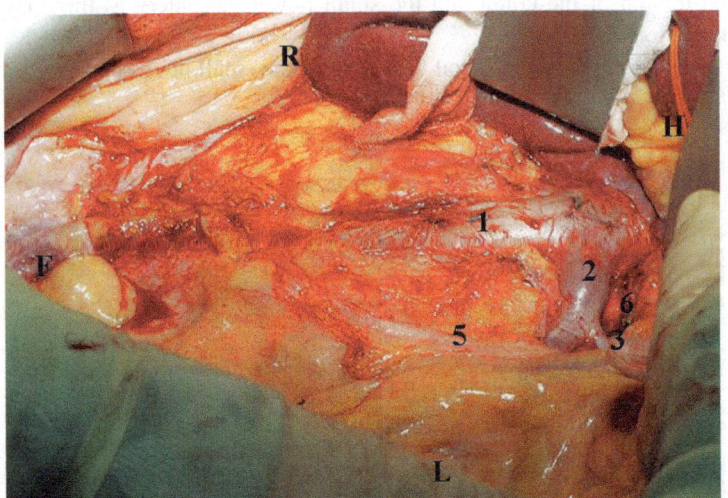

Fig. 5.11 The completed Cattel–Braasch and Kocher maneouver. 1 – IVC, 2 – Left renal vein, 3 – Left adrenal vein, 4 – Infrarenal aorta, 5 – IMV, 6 – abdominal aorta

The Cattel–Braasch (3) manoeuvre when completed gives you very good access to the entire retroperinoneum, with access to the following organs and structures:

- Abdominal aorta below the SMA
- IVC
- SMA

- Inferior mesenteric artery (IMA) and inferior mesenteric vein (IMV)
- Celiac trunk and plexus
- Both kidneys, renal veins and ureters
- Iliac vessels – both sides
- Posterior side of the duodenum and the pancreas head
- Left adrenal gland and the left adrenal vein (Fig. 5.11)

Literature

1. Hirshberg A, Mattox KL (2005). The crash laparotomy. In: H. Asher (ed.) The Top Knife the Art and Craft of Trauma Surgery, tfm Publishing Ltd, Castle Hill Barns, Harley, Shrewsbury Harely, 53–70
2. Skandalakis JE, Colborn GL, Weidman TA, Badalament RA, Parrot TS, Zoras O, Mirilas PS. (2004) Retroperitoneum. In: Skandalakis JE, Weidman TA, Foster Jr RS Jr, Kingsnorth AN, Skandalakis LJ, Skandalakis PN, Mirilas PS (editors.). Skandalakis' Surgical Anatomy. The Embryologic and Anatomic Basis of Modern Surgery, vol. I, Paschalidis Medical Publications Ltd., Athens, 2004, vol. I, 552–577
3. Cattel R, Braasch J (1960)., A technique for the exposure of the third and fourth portion of the duodenum., Surgery Gynaecological Obstetrics, 1960,11:, 379

Chapter 6
Infrarenal and Superior Mesenteric Artery Major Vessel Dissection

Abstract Background: Superior mesenteric artery (SMA) and infrarenal major vessel dissection is the next step after the Cattel–Braasch manoeuvre, which consists of dissection, in the retroperitonem, of the following vessels and structures: infrarenal aorta, inferior vena cava (IVC), SMA, inferior mesenteric artery (IMA), inferior mesenteric vein (IMV), celiac trunk and plexus and iliac vessels on both sides. Abdominal aorta and IVC are dissected and encircled close to their bifurcations with long, thick ligatures. The left renal vein after mobilisation is encircled with the vessel loop. During the retroperitoneum inspection, special attention has to be paid to the quality of the abdominal aorta and any vascular abnormality.

Conclusion: SMA and infrarenal major vessel dissection and retroperitoneum inspection are some of the most important steps before aorta and IVC cannulation.

Keywords Aorta, Inferior vena cava, Superior mesenteric artery, Infrarenal major vessels dissection

6.1 Abdominal Aorta and Inferior Vena Cava

6.1.1 Surgical Steps

1. With the right angulated clamp, free the abdominal aorta and inferior vena cava (IVC) from their bifurcations up to the liver and the superior mesenteric artery (SMA).
2. Palpate the abdominal aorta, IVC, common external iliac arteries. Check for state of arteriosclerosis (Fig. 6.1), and/or an aberrant low (Fig. 6.2) or in front of IVC running right aberrant renal artery or arteries (Fig. 6.3).
3. Cut and ligate the inferior mesenteric vein (IMV) (Figs. 6.4 and 6.5), on the left side of Treitz ligament. This manoeuvre will give you good access later to the celiac plexus, left renal and left adrenal veins (Fig. 6.6).

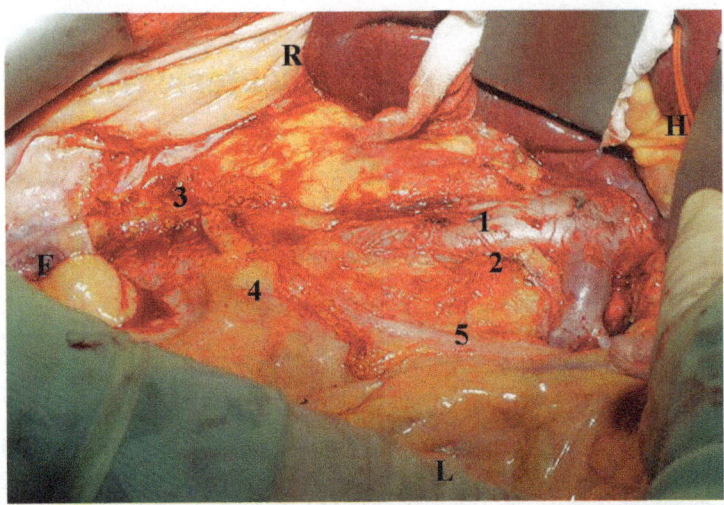

Fig. 6.1 1 – Inferior vena cava (IVC), 2 – Abdominal aorta, 3 – Right common iliac artery, 4 – Left common iliac artery, 5 – Inferior mesenteric vein (IMV), *H – head, F – feet, R – right, L – left*

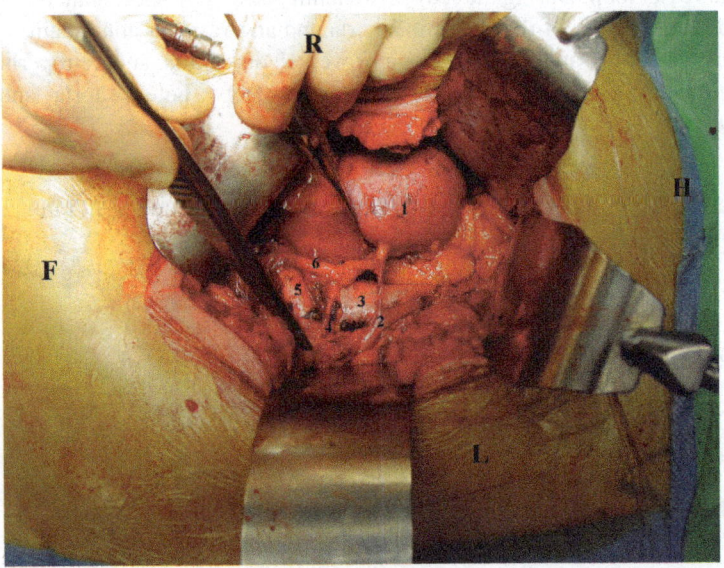

Fig. 6.2 Accessory renal artery. 1 – Right kidney, 2 – Right gonadal vein, 3 – IVC, 4 – Right accessory renal artery arising from right common iliac artery, 5 – Common iliac artery, 6 – right ureter, *H – head, F – feet, R – right, L – left*

6.1 Abdominal Aorta and Inferior Vena Cava

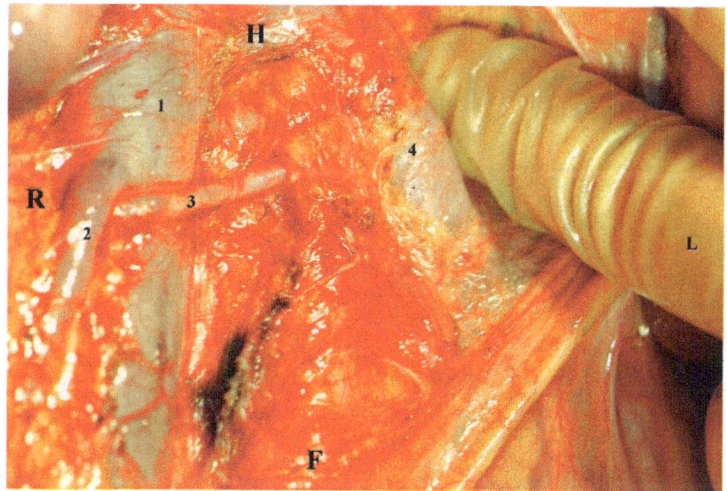

Fig. 6.3 Right accessory renal artery. 1 – IVC, 2 – Right gonadal vein, 3 – Right accessory renal artery running in front of IVC, 4 – Aorta, *H – head, F – feet, R – right, L – left*

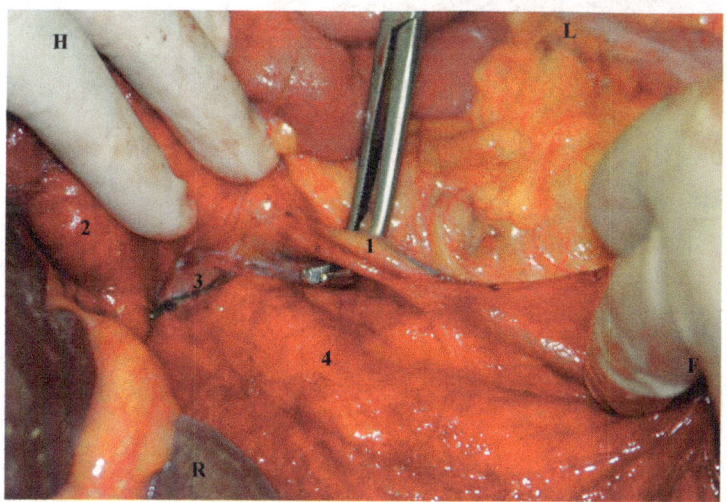

Fig. 6.4 1 – IMV, 2 – Duodenum, 3 – Left renal vein, 4 – Abdominal aorta, *H – head, F – feet, R – right, L – left*

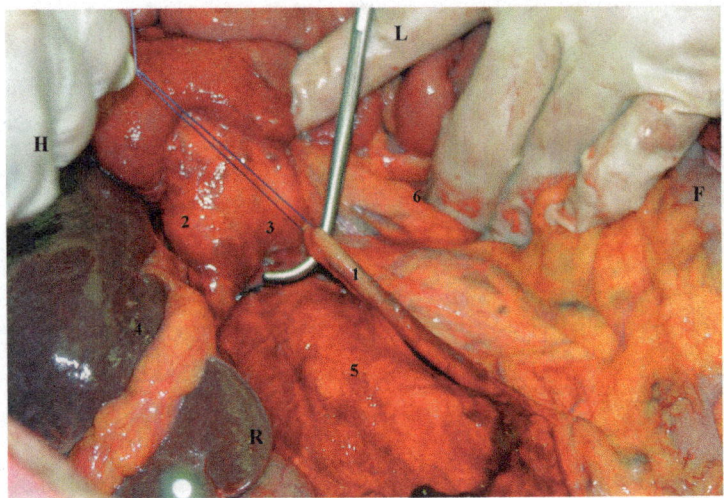

Fig. 6.5 1 – Ligated IMV, 2 – Duodenum, 3 – Pancreas head posterior side, 4 – Liver, 5 – Abdominal aorta colon, 6 – Pancreas tail, *H – head, F – feet, R – right, L – left*

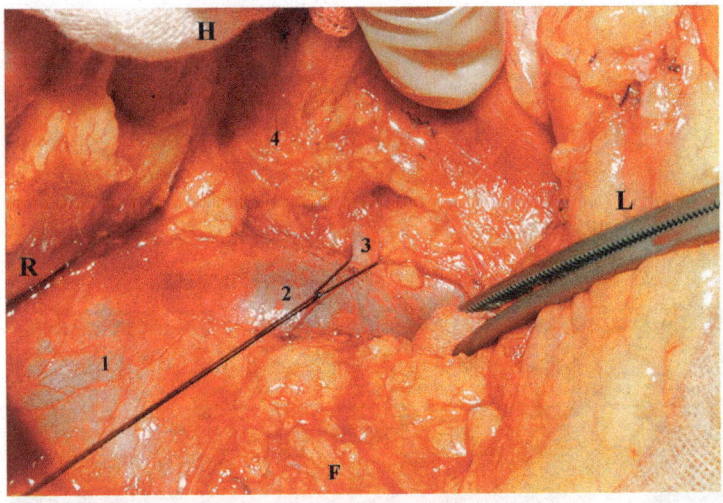

Fig. 6.6 1 – IVC, 2 – Left renal vein, 3 – Left adrenal vein, 4 – Celiac plexus, *H – head, F – feet, R – right, L – left*

4. Mobilise the left renal vein, dissect and mobilise the inferior mesenteric artery (IMA) (Fig. 6.7).
5. Dissect and encircle the abdominal aorta (Fig. 6.8) and IVC (Fig. 6.9), each with two long, thick ligatures (no. 2) close to their bifurcation (Fig. 6.10).

6.1 Abdominal Aorta and Inferior Vena Cava

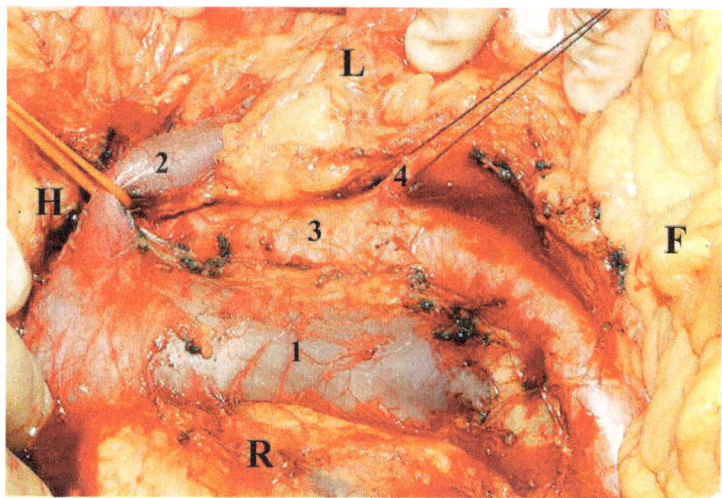

Fig. 6.7 1 – IVC, 2 – Mobilised left renal vein, 3 – Abdominal aorta, 4 – Mobilised inferior mesenteric artery (IMA), *H – head, F – feet, R – right, L – left*

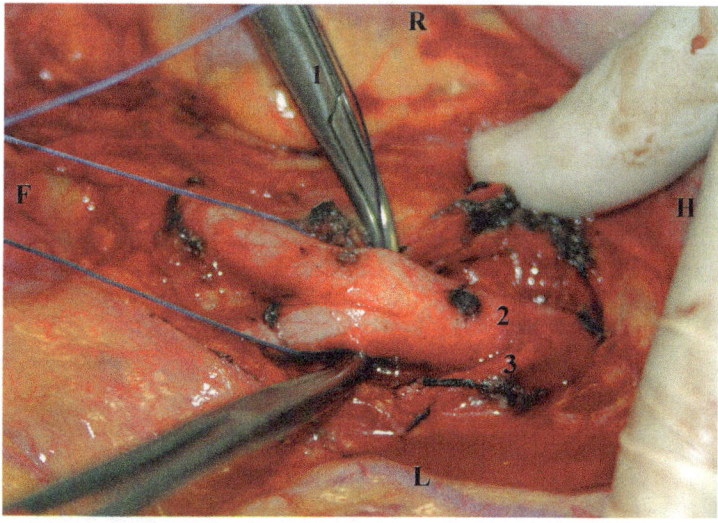

Fig. 6.8 1 – Angulated clamp, 2 – Abdominal aorta, 3 – IMA, *H – head, F – feet, R – right, L – left*

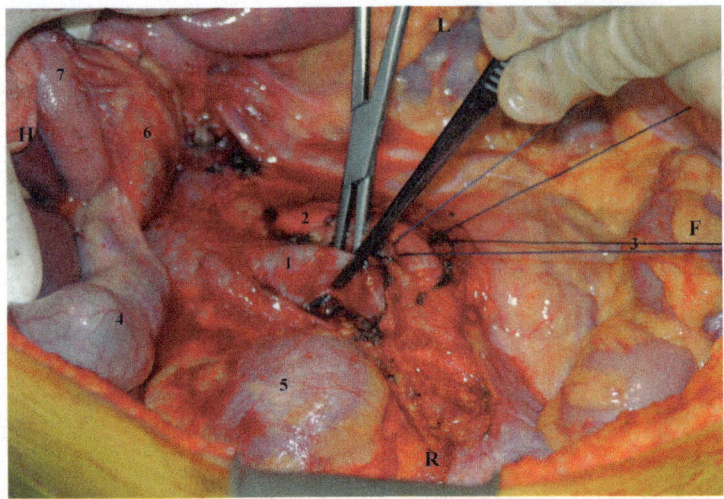

Fig. 6.9 1 – IVC, 2 – Abdominal aorta, 3 – Thick, strong ligatures, 4 – Gallbladder, 5 – Right kidney, 6 – Pancreas head posterior part, 7 – Duodenum, *H – head, F – feet, R – right, L – left*

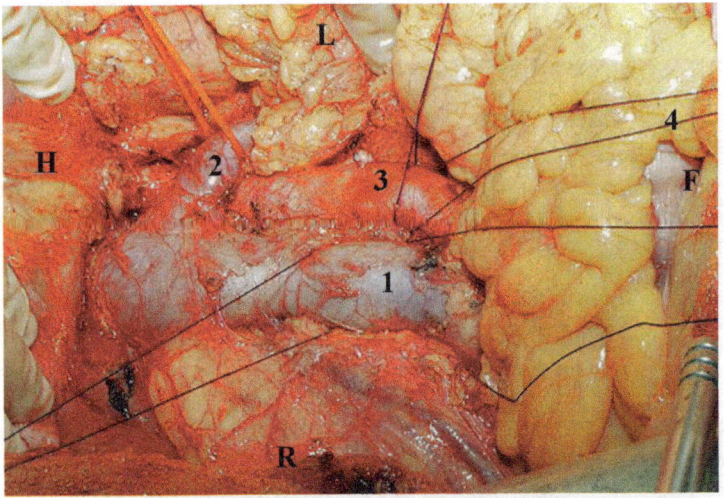

Fig. 6.10 1 – IVC, 2 – Left renal vein, 3 – Abdominal aorta, 4 – Ligature placed around the abdominal aorta, *H – head, F – feet, R – right, L – left*

6. Beyond the abdominal cavity, fixate each ligature with separate clamp (Fig. 6.11).

ATTENTION!
- If there is a lower pole kidney artery originating from the iliac vessel, cannulation of one of the iliac external artery must be considered (Fig. 6.3).

6.1 Abdominal Aorta and Inferior Vena Cava

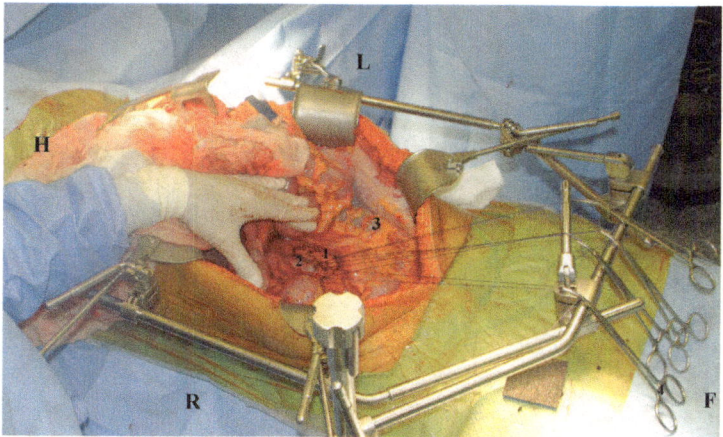

Fig. 6.11 1 – Abdominal aorta, 2 – IVC, 3 – Sigmoid, 4 – Separate clamp, *H – head, F – feet, R – right, L – left*

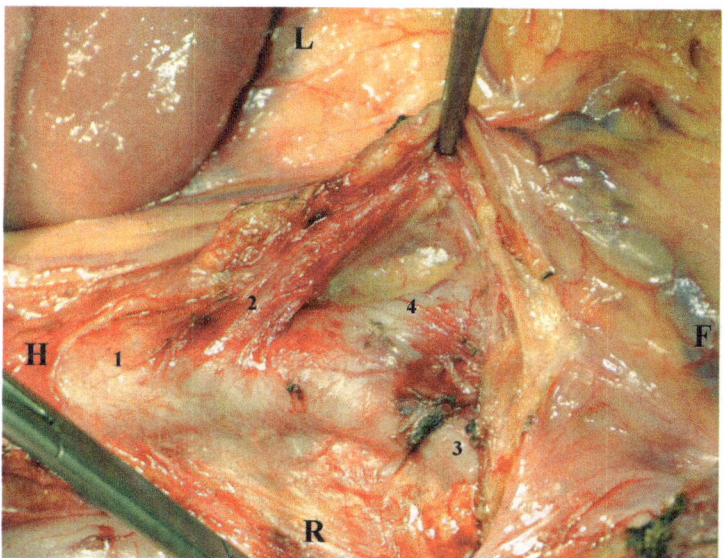

Fig. 6.12 1 – Abdominal aorta, 2 – IMA, 3 – Right common iliac artery, 4 – Left common iliac artery, *H – head, F – feet, R – right, L – left*

- Look at the distance between the IMA and the aorta's bifurcation (Fig. 6.12). If the distance is too small (Fig. 6.13), and the cannulation of the aorta can be difficult, ligate and cut the IMA (Fig. 6.14).
- If because of severe arteriosclerosis, aneurysm or any other reason abdominal aorta cannulation is impossible, dissect the common and external iliac artery – palpate and choose which the best side for cannulation is.

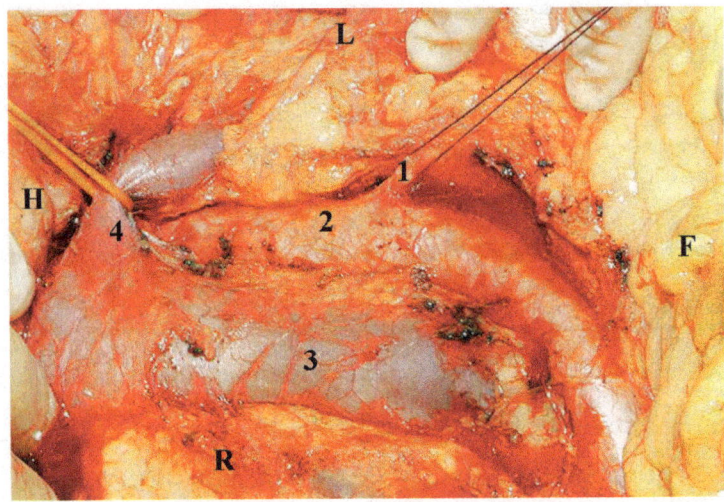

Fig. 6.13 Very short distance between AMI and aorta's bifurcation. 1 – IMA before ligation, 2 – Abdominal aorta, 3 – IVC, *H – head, F – feet, R – right, L – left*

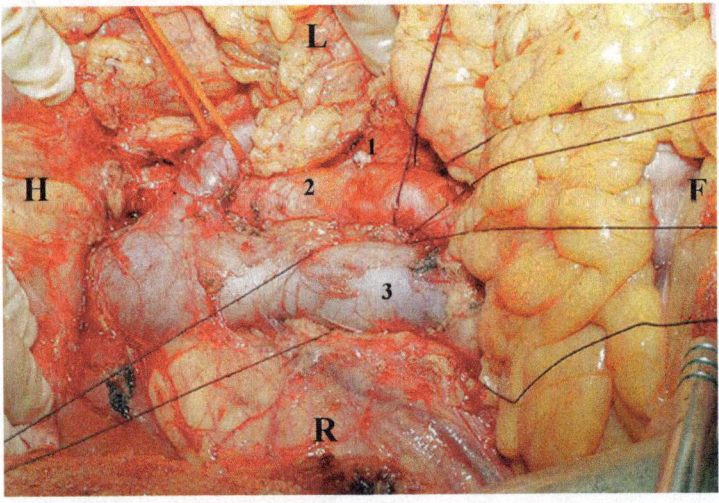

Fig. 6.14 Short distance between IMA and aorta's bifurcation. 1 – Ligated IMA, 2 – Abdominal aorta, 3 – IVC, *H – head, F – feet, R – right, L – left*

- If the cannulation is still difficult, dissect, ligate and cut off distally one of the less arteriosclerotic iliac external arteries. Total iliac external artery mobilisation will make cannulation much easier.
- If the cannulation of the iliac vessels is impossible consider retrograde cannulation from the aorta below the diaphragm or left subclavian artery (1).

6.1 Abdominal Aorta and Inferior Vena Cava

- If the cannulation from the aorta arch is also impossible, after donor full heparinisation choose one of the rapid procurement techniques and flush the procured organs during bench procedure (2–5).

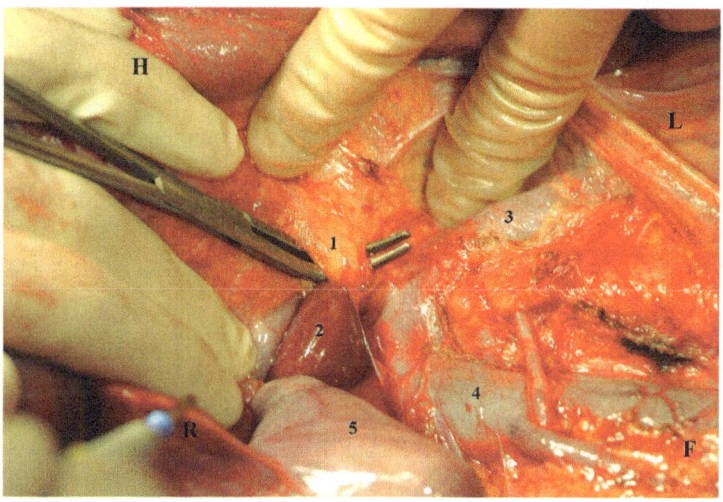

Fig. 6.15 Superior mesenteric artery (SMA) dissection. 1 – Celiac plexus, 2 – Caudate lobe of the liver, 3 – Left renal vein, 4 – IVC, 5 – Gallbladder, *H – head, F – feet, R – right, L – left*

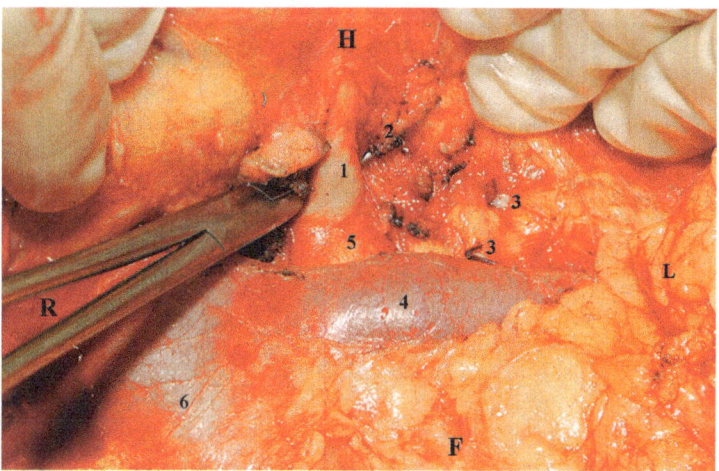

Fig. 6.16 Dissected SMA. 1 – SMA, 2 – Dissected celiac plexus, 3 – Ligated and cut left adrenal vein, 4 – Left renal vein, 5 – Abdominal aorta, 6 – IVC, *H – head, F – feet, R – right, L – left*

6.2 Superior Mesenteric Artery

6.2.1 Surgical Steps

1. With angulated clamp, dissect the celiac plexus around SMA up to 1.5 cm from the abdominal aorta (Fig. 6.15).

ATTENTION!
- If the access to the SMA is difficult, cut and ligate the left adrenal vein (Fig. 6.16).
- Look for the right aberrant accessory or replaced (common) hepatic artery arising from the SMA.
- Avoid damage of the pancreatoduodenal trunk arising from the SMA or the renal arteries. Remember that in most cases they are at the level of SMA or just below, but in a few cases, renal arteries could be arising above the SMA (6, 7).

Literature

1. Molmenti EE, Molmenti P, Molmenti H et al (2001) Cannulation of the aorta in organ donors with infrarenal pathologies, Digestieve Diseases and Science: 46(11): 2457–2459
2. Nakazato PZ, Conception W, Limm W et al (1993) Total abdominal evisceration: an en bloc technique for abdominal organ harvesting, Surgery: 111: 37–47
3. Nghiem DD (1996) Rapid exenteration for multiorgan harvesting: a new technique for the unstable donor, Transplant Proceeding: 28: 256–257
4. Pinna AD, Dodson FS, Smith CV et al (1997) Rapid en bloc technique for liver and pancreas procurement, Transplant Proceeding: 29: 647–648
5. Imagawa DK, Olthoff KM, Yerzis H et al (1996) Rapid en bloc technique for pancreas-liver procurement, Transplantation: 61: 1605–1609
6. Brockman JG, Vaidya A, Reddy S et al (2006) Retrival of abdominal organs for transplantation, British Journal of Surgery: 93: 113–146
7. Skandalakis JE, Colborn GL, Weidman TA, Badalament RA, Parrot TS, Zoras O, Mirilas PS (2004) Retroperitoneum. In Skandalakis JE, Weidman TA, Foster RS Jr, Kingsnorth AN, Skandalakis LJ, Skandalakis PN, Mirilas PS (eds.) Skandalakis' Surgical Anatomy. The Embryologic and Anatomic Basis of Modern Surgery, Vol. I, Paschalidis Medical Publications, Athens, 552–577

Chapter 7
Left Liver Lobe and Supraceliac Aorta

Abstract Background: Placing the bowels in the physiological position in the abdomen, mobilisation of the left liver lobe, followed by lesser omentum inspection (left aberrant hepatic artery), abdominal oesophagus dissection and cutting the right crus of the diaphragm are the steps that have to be taken to access the supraceliac abdominal aorta. Freed and marked, the supraceliac aorta will be cross-clamped with a clamp or ligated with ligature during cold perfusion.

Conclusion: Freeing the abdominal aorta beneath diaphragm is necessary in order to perform aorta cross-clamping and start abdominal cold organ perfusion. Here, special attention must be paid to the presence of the left aberrant hepatic artery, which has to be saved.

Keywords Left liver lobe, Left triangular ligament, Supraceliac aorta dissection

7.1 Preparation

7.1.1 Colon and Small Bowel

1. Place the colon and the small bowel in the physiological position back into to the abdominal cavity (Fig. 7.1).

ATTENTION!
- During upper abdomen dissection, pay particular attention to blood perfusion of the abdominal organs and especially to the repositioned small bowel and the colon.
- Avoid bowel mesentery torsion. Restricted flow can cause ischemia.

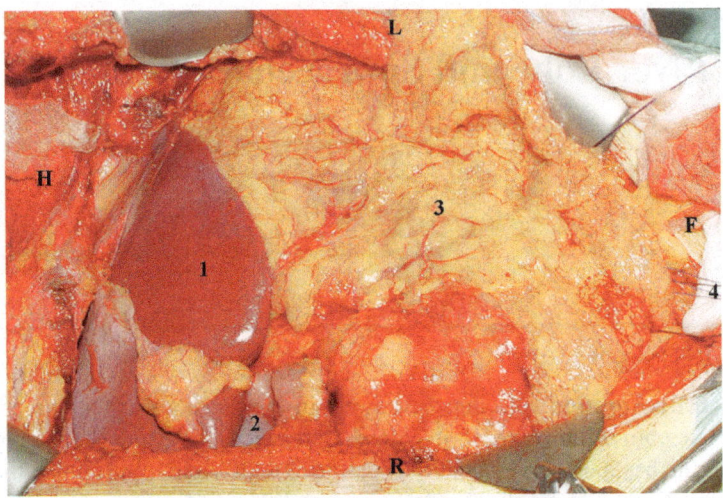

Fig. 7.1 Abdominal organs in the physiological position. 1 – Liver, 2 – Gallbladder, 3 – Greater omentum, 4 – Ligatures placed around the aorta and the IVC, *H – head, F – feet, R – right, L – left*

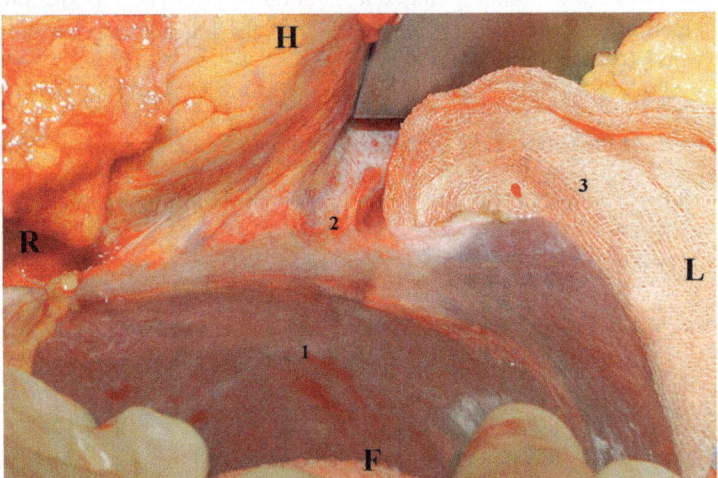

Fig. 7.2 Mobilisation of the left liver lobe. 1 – Left liver lobe, 2 – Left triangular ligament, 3 – Gauze, *H – head, F – feet, R – right, L – left*

7.2 Left Liver Lobe Mobilisation

7.2.1 Surgical Steps

1. Mobilise the left liver lobe by cutting the left triangular ligament (Fig. 7.2).

7.2 Left Liver Lobe Mobilisation

ATTENTION!
- In some cases, the left triangular ligament comes up or behind the spleen. Be careful to avoid bleeding because of spleen damage.

HOW TO DO IT:

Place a wet, warm gauze under the left liver lobe, behind the left triangular ligament (Fig. 7.3) and with another wet warm gauze, pull down the left liver lobe (Fig. 7.4). Put the light of the operating room on the left triangular ligament – the gauze will be shining through the ligament.

The gauze will protect the abdominal oesophagus, stomach and spleen from damage. Use the electrocautery to cut the ligament and free the left liver lobe (Figs. 7.5 and 7.6). Avoid damage of liver parenchyma, left inferior phrenic and left hepatic veins.

2. Gently place the left liver lobe to the right side using the hand of the assistant (Fig. 7.7) or blade of a professional abdominal retractor (Fig. 7.10).
3. Inspect the lesser omentum (hepatogastric ligament) for the presence of a left aberrant (accessory or replaced) hepatic artery (Fig. 7.8).

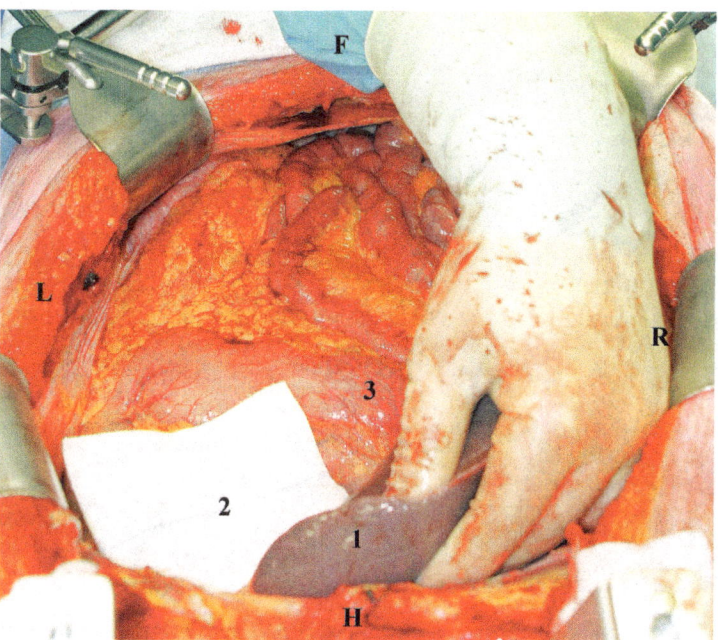

Fig. 7.3 1 – Left liver lobe, 2 – Warm, wet gauze under the left liver lobe, 3 – Stomach, *H – head, F – feet, R – right, L – left*

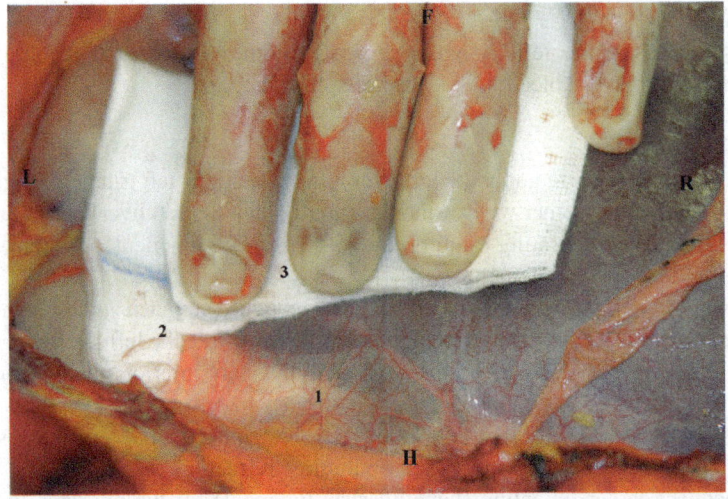

Fig. 7.4 1 – Left triangular ligament, 2 – Warm, wet gauze under the left triangular ligament, 3 – The second warm, wet gauze on the left liver lobe, *H – head, F – feet, R – right, L – left*

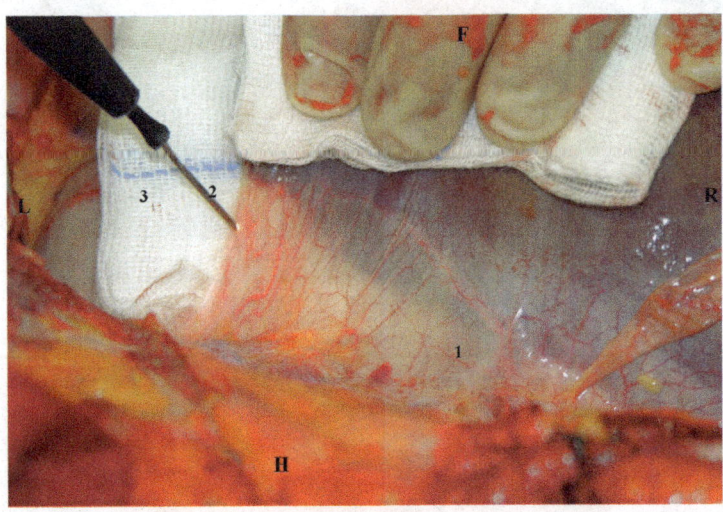

Fig. 7.5 1 – Left triangular ligament, 2 – Electrocautery, 3 – Gauze under left liver lobe, *H – head, F – feet, R – right, L – left*

7.2 Left Liver Lobe Mobilisation

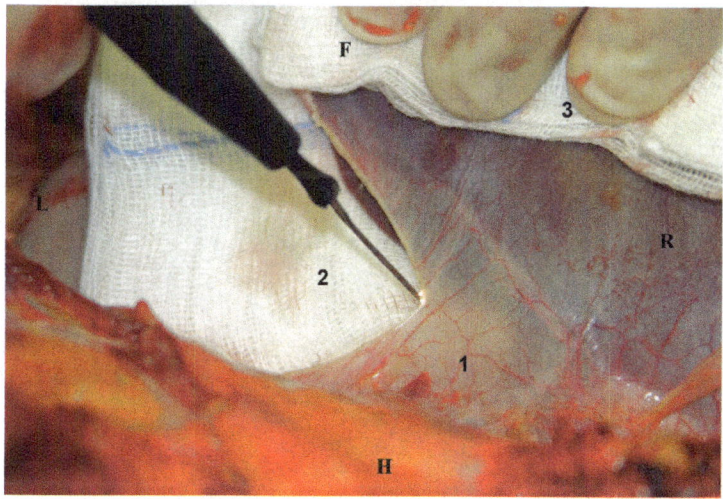

Fig. 7.6 1 – Left triangular ligament, 2 – Gauze under the left liver lobe, 3 – The second gauze on the left liver lobe, *H – head, F – feet, R – right, L – left*

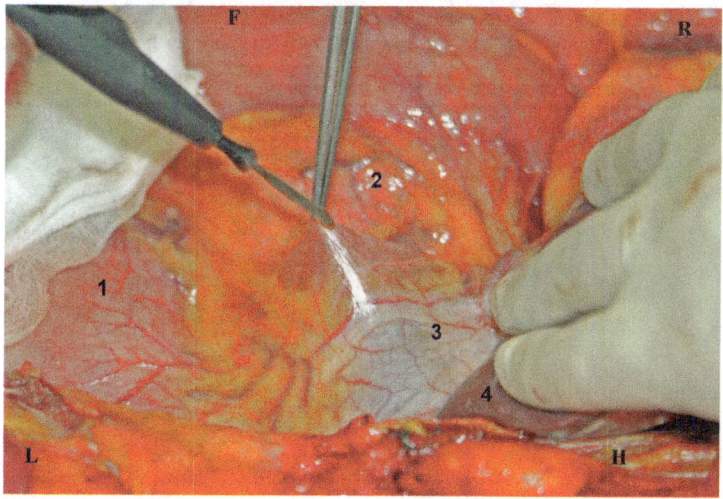

Fig. 7.7 1 – Stomach, 2 – Pancreas, 3 – Lesser omentum, 4 – Left liver lobe, *H – head, F – feet, R – right, L – left*

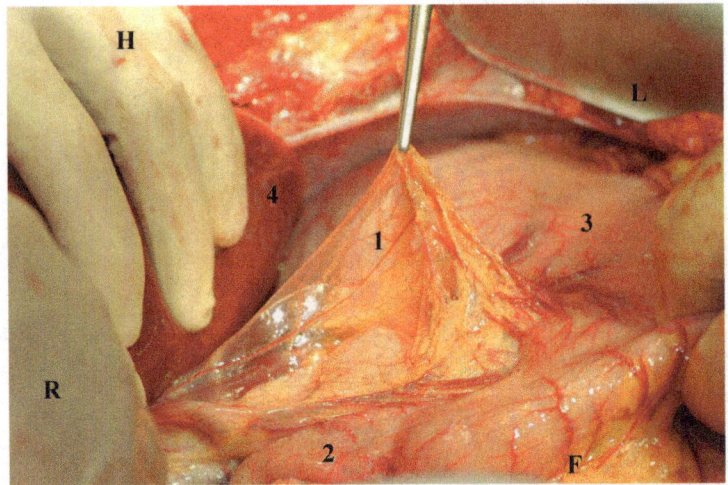

Fig. 7.8 Hepatogastric ligament inspection. 1 – Lesser omentum, 2 – Duodenum, 3 – Stomach, 4 – Left liver lobe, *H – head, F – feet, R – right, L – left*

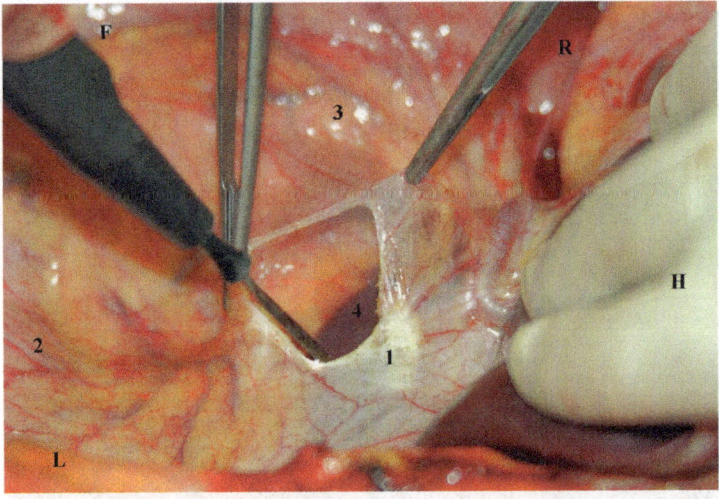

Fig. 7.9 1 – Lesser omentum, 2 – Stomach, 3 – Pancreas, 4 – Caudate liver lobe, *H – head, F – feet, R – right, L – left*

ATTENTION!

- If there is no left aberrant hepatic artery cut the lesser omentum with electrocautery, from the diaphragm up to the hepatoduodenal ligament – black broken line (Figs. 7.9 and 7.10).

7.2 Left Liver Lobe Mobilisation

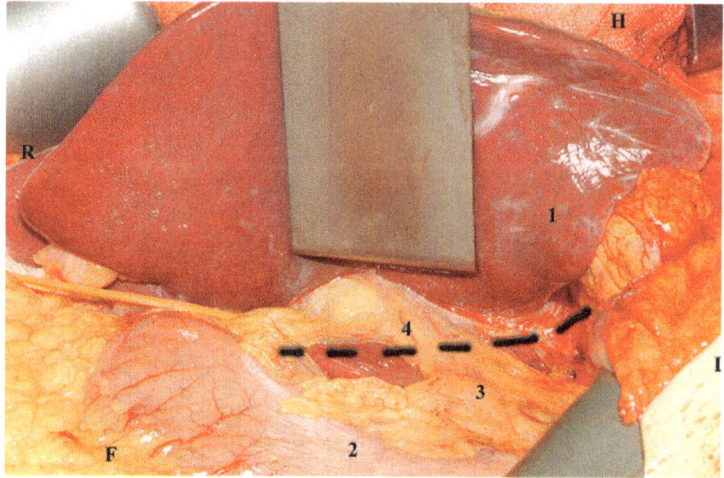

Fig. 7.10 1 – Left liver lobe, 2 – Stomach, 3 – Lesser omentum, 4 – Line of cutting lesser omentum, if there is no left aberrant hepatic artery present the black broken line indicate the line of dissection, *H – head, F – feet, R – right, L – left*

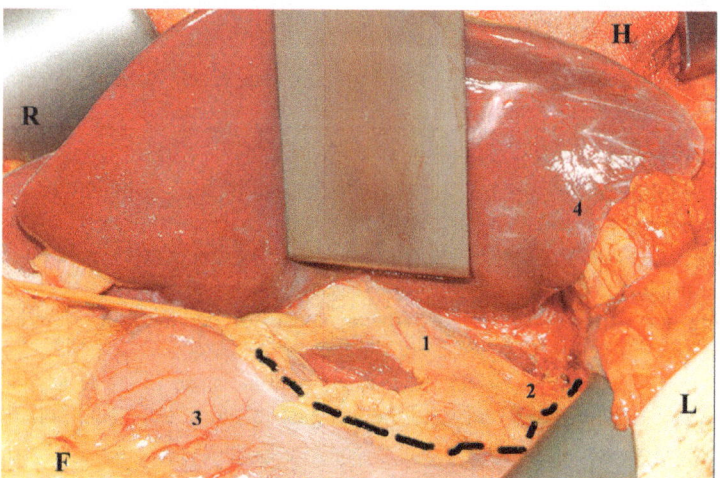

Fig. 7.11 The black broken line indicates the line of incision of the lower lesser omentum if the left aberrant hepatic artery is present. 1 – Left aberrant hepatic artery, 2 – Lesser omentum, 3 – Stomach, 4 – Left liver lobe, *H – head, F – feet, R – right, L – left* (remember: it is better and safer to do this after organ perfusion)

- If there is a left aberrant hepatic artery, save it by mobilising the lesser omentum, close to the stomach, after cold organ perfusion (Fig. 7.11). During inspection be very careful to avoid haematoma. *Remember–* the smallest haematoma can prevent sufficient perfusion of the liver and thus cause damage to the intrahepatic biliary tree.

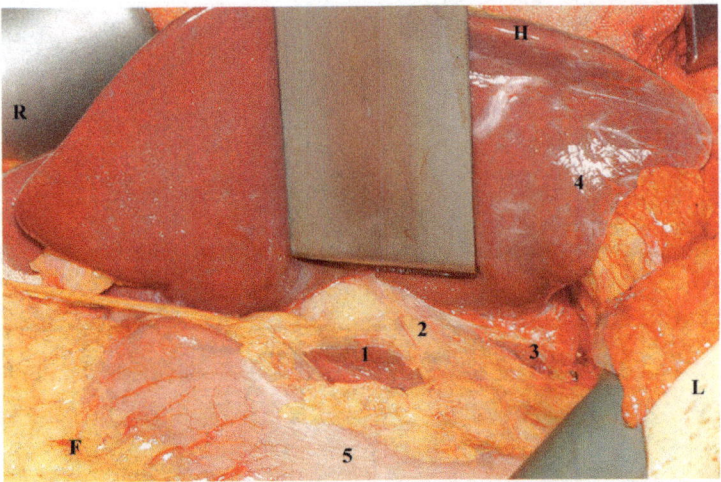

Fig. 7.12 1 – Divided lesser omentum beneath the left aberrant hepatic artery, 2 – Left aberrant hepatic artery, 3 – Divided lesser omentum above the left aberrant hepatic artery, 4 – Left liver lobe, *H – head, F – feet, R – right, L – left*

- When there is only one replaced, left hepatic artery, pay critical attention to its preservation.

HOW TO DO IT – step by step:
- After mobilisation of the left liver lobe, pull the stomach very gently downwards.
- Divide, with electrocautery, the hepatogastric ligament 2–3 cm beneath and above the left aberrant hepatic artery (Fig. 7.12).
- During aorta dissection, avoid damage, spasm or haematoma around the left aberrant hepatic artery.
- After organ perfusion, dissect the lesser omentum close to the lesser curvature of the stomach wall together with the left gastric and left aberrant hepatic arteries, up to the diaphragm.

7.3 Visualisation of the Abdominal Aorta Beneath the Diaphragm

7.3.1 Surgical Steps

1. Free the abdominal part of the oesophagus, encircle with tape and pull it to the left side of the abdomen (Fig. 7.13).

7.3 Visualisation of the Abdominal Aorta Beneath the Diaphragm

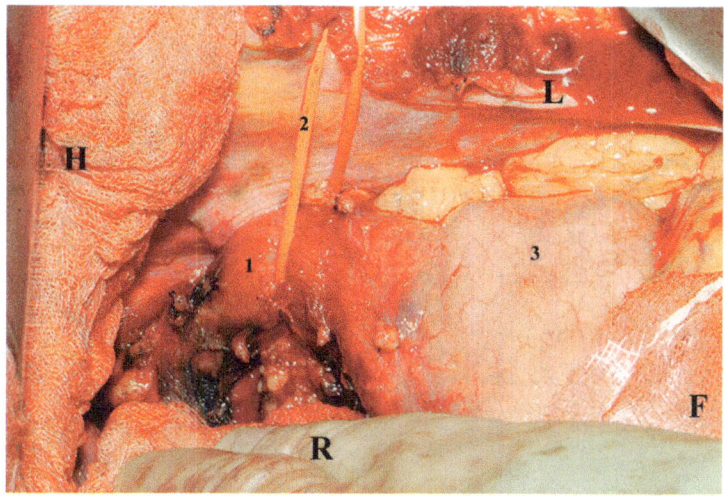

Fig. 7.13 Dissected oesophagus. 1 – Oesophagus, 2 – Tape, 3 – Stomach, *H – head, F – feet, R – right, L – left*

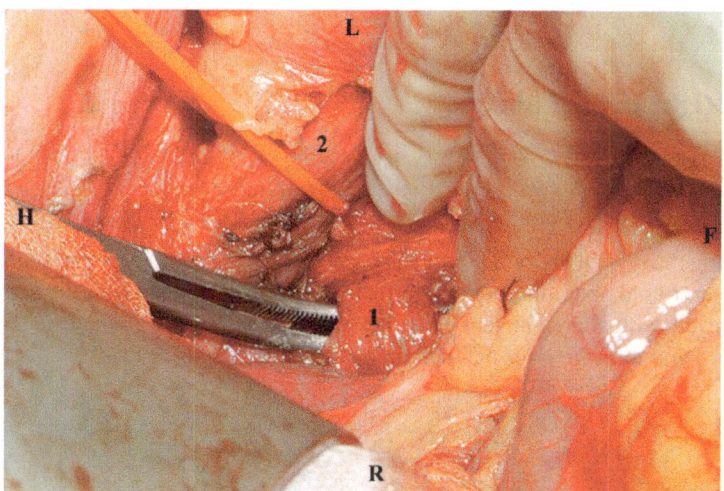

Fig. 7.14 1 – Right crus of the diaphragm, 2 – Oesophagus, *H – head, F – feet, R – right, L – left*

2. Divide the right crus of the diaphragm from the aortic hiatus up to the celiac trunk (Fig. 7.14).
3. Free and encircle the abdominal aorta under the diaphragm with a long thick ligature Vicryl (Ethicon) no. 2 or mark it with the long tape (Fig. 7.15).

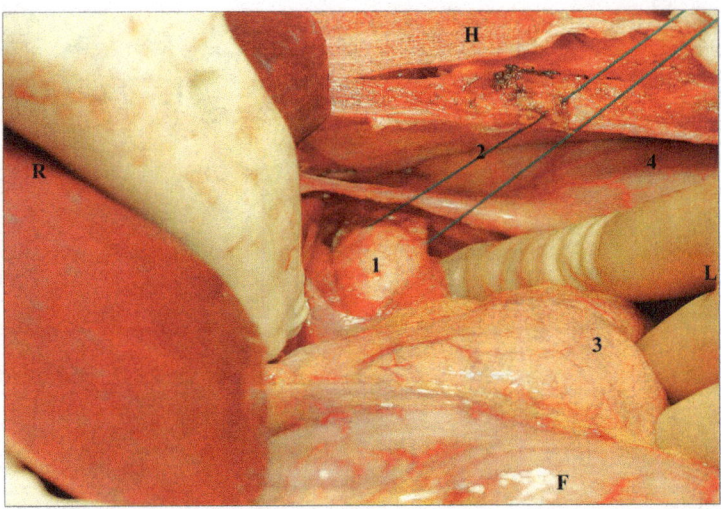

Fig. 7.15 Freed supraceliac abdominal aorta. 1 – Abdominal aorta under the diaphragm, 2 – Thick ligature, 3 – Pancreas, 4 – Stomach, *H – head, F – feet, R – right, L – left*

7.4 Right Liver Lobe

7.4.1 Surgical Steps

1. During the typical abdominal organ procurement the right liver lobe is mobilised just after cold abdominal organ perfusion. The liver and the right liver lobe are retrieved with the right leaflet of the diaphragm. This technique is safe and allows you to avoid liver parenchyma iatrogenic injury.

Chapter 8
Hepatoduodenal Ligament and Biliary Tree

Abstract Background: The hepatoduodenal ligament extends between the liver and the first portion of the duodenum and is continuous with the right border of the hepatogastric ligament. It contains the common bile duct, hepatic artery and portal vein as well as the hepatic plexus and the lymph nodes.

Recognising abnormal arterial vascularisation and creating the *landmarks* (small segment dissection) of the following structures: common bile duct (CBD), gastroduodenal artery and common, proper and/or aberrant hepatic artery are very important steps during abdominal organ procurement. Flushing the CBD, intrahepatic biliary tree and cleaning the gallbladder or ligating of cystic duct will prevent intra-hepatic biliary lesions after liver transplantation.

Conclusion: Creating landmarks by partial dissection of the hepatoduodenal ligament structures before organ perfusion is very important and could have an important influence on the quality and transplantability of the pancreas and the liver.

Keywords Hepatoduodenal ligament, Biliary tree, Gastroduodenal artery, Portal vein aberrant right hepatic artery, Common bile duct, Gallbladder

8.1 Definition, Ligament Inspection and Dissection

8.1.1 Definition

The hepatoduodenal ligament extends between the liver and the first portion of the duodenum and is continuous with the right border of the hepatogastric ligament. It contains the common bile duct, hepatic artery and portal vein as well as the hepatic plexus and the lymph nodes (1) (Fig. 8.1).

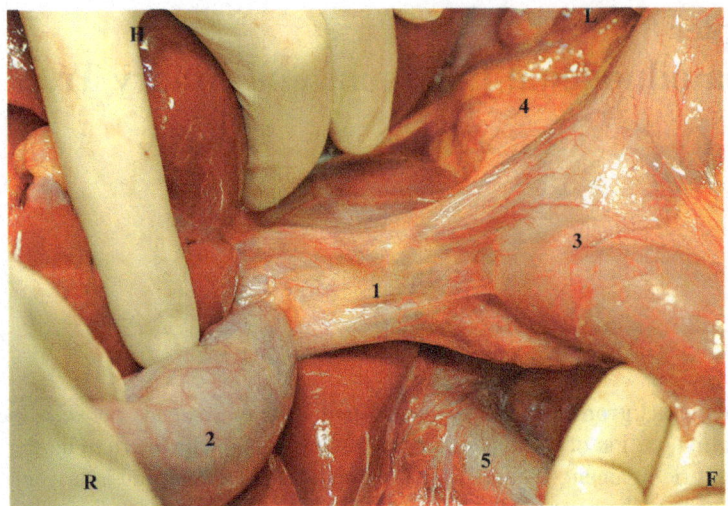

Fig. 8.1 1 – Hepatoduodenal ligament, 2 – Gallbladder, 3 – Duodenum, 4 – Pancreas, 5 – IVC, H – head, F – feet, R – right, L – left

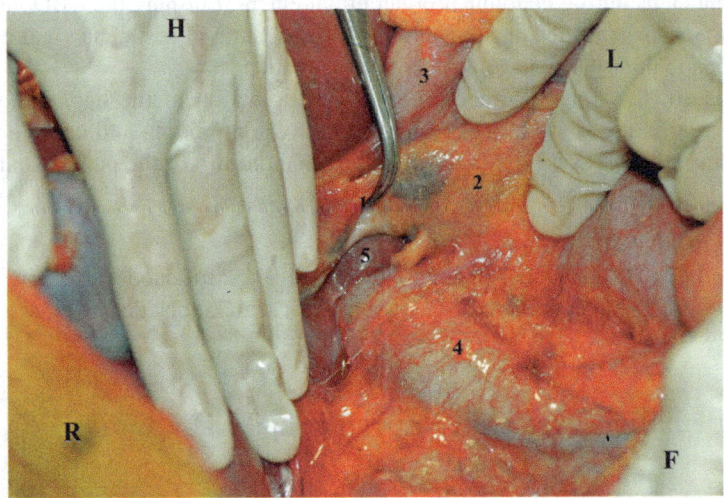

Fig. 8.2 1 – Posterior side of the hepatoduodenal ligament, 2 – Posterior side of the pancreas head, 3 – Duodenum, 4 – IVC, 5 – caudate lobe of the liver, H – head, F – feet, R – right, L – left

8.1.2 *Hepatoduodenal Ligament Inspection: In Steps*

1. Gently lift up the duodenum and the head of the pancreas together with the hepatoduodenal ligament (Fig. 8.2).

8.1 Definition, Ligament Inspection and Dissection 77

2. Examine the posterior side of the hepatoduodenal ligament. Look for the right aberrant hepatic artery arising from the SMA (Fig. 8.3 – accessory hepatic artery and Fig. 8.4 – replaced hepatic artery).

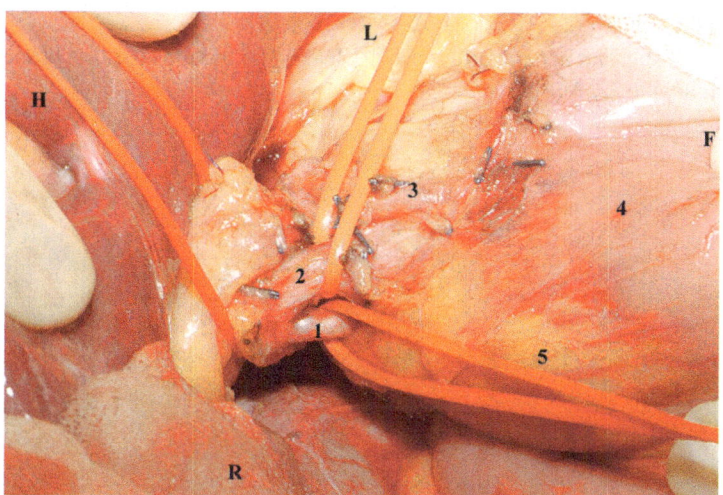

Fig. 8.3 1 – Right aberrant hepatic artery (accessory), 2 – Common bile duct, 3 – Gastroduodenal artery, 4 – Stomach, 5 – Posterior side of the pancreas head, *H – head, F – feet, R – right, L – left*

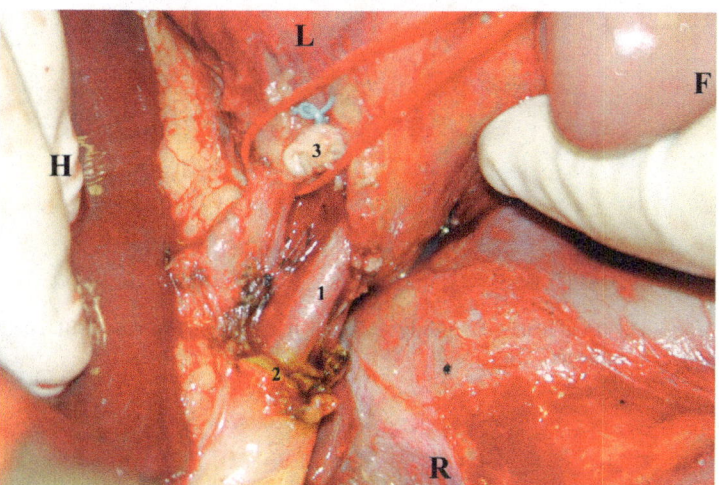

Fig. 8.4 1 – Right aberrant hepatic artery (replaced), 2 – The incised proximal part of the common bile duct, 3 – Ligated distal part of the common bile duct, *H – head, F – feet, R – right, L – left*

3. The presence of this artery can be detected by palpating or gently squeezing the hepatoduodenal ligament between the thumb and the index finger (under the common bile duct on the right side or behind the portal vein) (Fig. 8.5).
4. If present, try to recognize it and inform the transplant coordinator, the liver and pancreas acceptor centre.

ATTENTION!
- The right aberrant hepatic artery usually leaves the SMA as the first branch from the right side (2, 3).

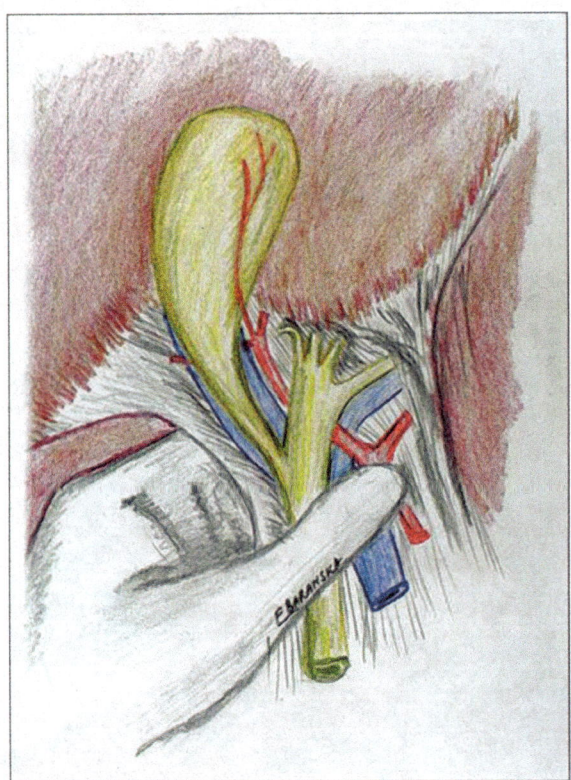

Fig. 8.5 Hepatoduodenal ligament – gently squeezing the common bile duct (CBD) between the thumb and the index finger

8.2 The Common Bile Duct (CBD) Dissection

8.2.1 Surgical Steps

1. Identify the CBD above the pancreas head and free 1.5 cm of it (Fig. 8.6).
2. Mark the CBD with the vessel loop (Fig. 8.7).

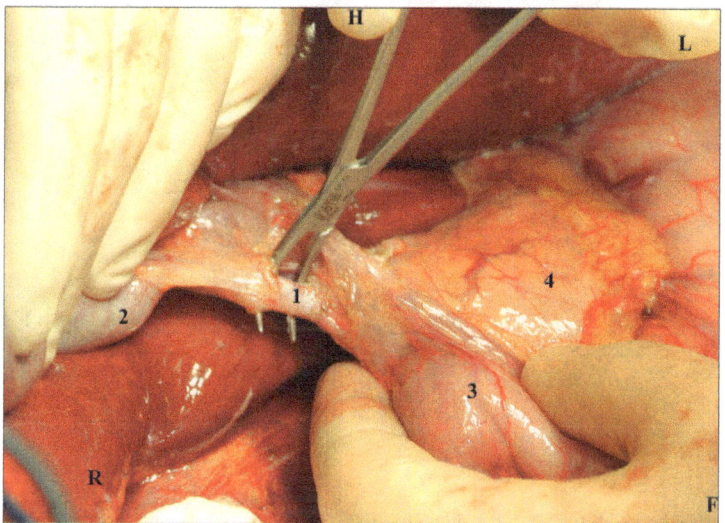

Fig. 8.6 1 – Common bile duct, 2 – Gallbladder, 3 – Duodenum, 4 – Pancreas, *H – head, F – feet, R – right, L – left*

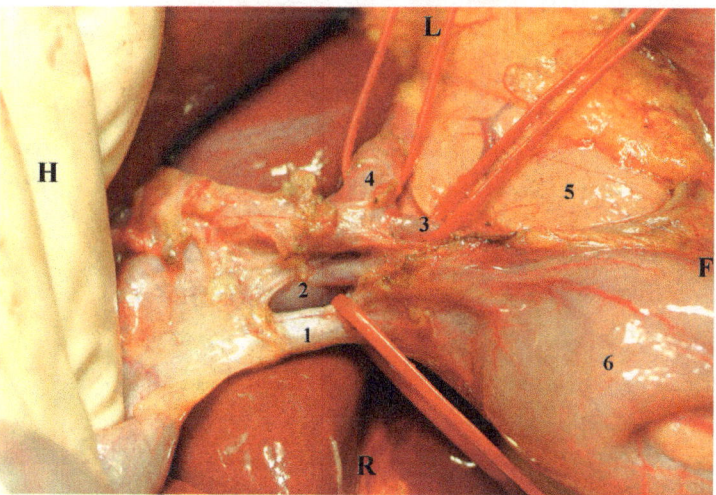

Fig. 8.7 CBD marked with vessel loop. 1 – CBD, 2 – Portal vein, 3 – Gastroduodenal artery, 4 – Common hepatic artery, 5 – Pancreas head, 6 – Duodenum, *H – head, F – feet, R – right, L – left*

3. Close to the pancreas head, ligate the distal part of the CBD and cut it with scissors (Figs. 8.8 and 8.9).
4. Flush (under low-pressure) the common bile duct and the intrahepatic biliary tree. Make use of about 300 mL of warm Ringer solution (Fig. 8.10).

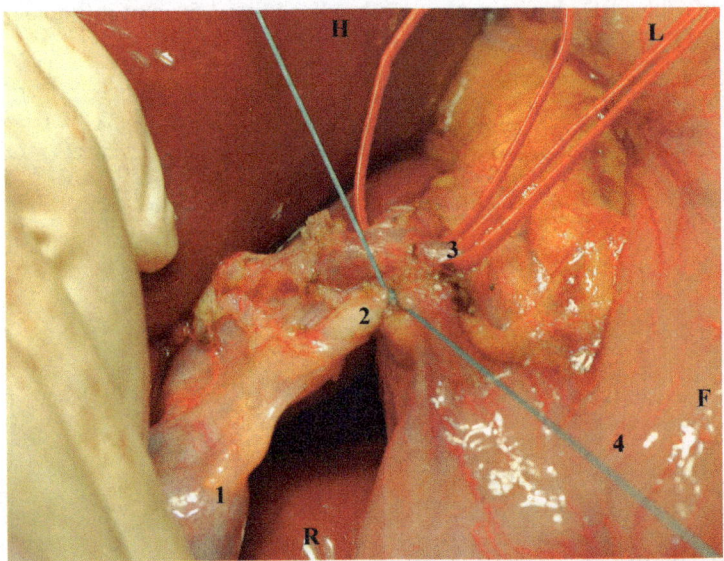

Fig. 8.8 Ligated CBD. 1– Gallbladder, 2 – CBD, 3 – Gastroduodenal artery, 4 – Stomach, H – head, F – feet, R – right, L – left

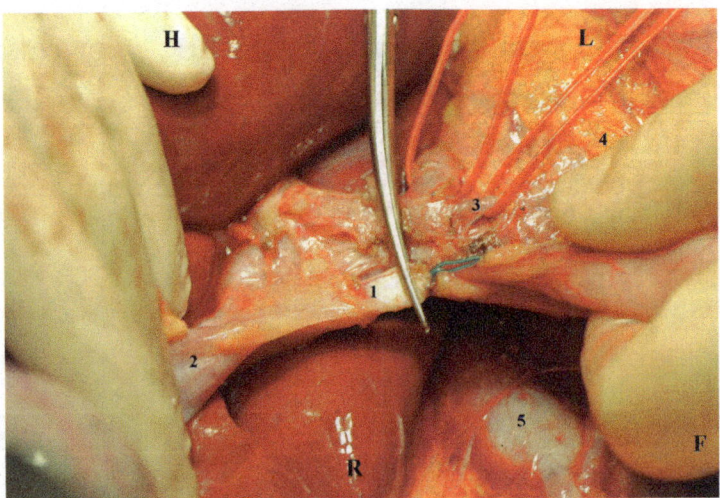

Fig. 8.9 1 – Ligated and cutting CBD, 2 – Gallbladder, 3 – Gastroduodenal artery, 4 – Pancreas, H – head, F – feet, R – right, L – left

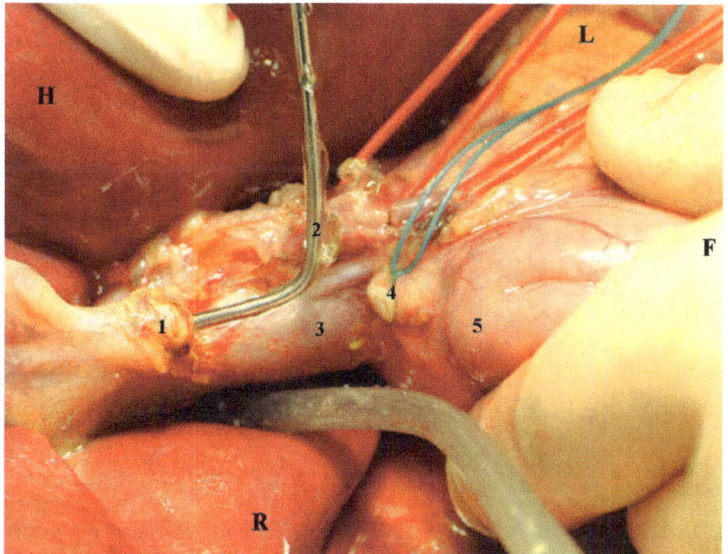

Fig. 8.10 1 – Proximal part of the CBD, 2 – Flushing the CBD under low pressure, 3 – Portal vein, 4 – Ligated and cut distal CBD, 5 – Duodenum, *H – head, F – feet, R – right, L – left*

8.3 The Gallbladder

8.3.1 Possibilities of Treatment: In Steps

1. Opening of the gallbladder - open the gallbladder; use the suction to evacuate the gall (Figs. 8.11 and 8.12), wash the gallbladder thoroughly with sterile Ringer or 0.9% NaCl solution. Use about 300 mL in total, as the gallbladder has to be free of bile (Figs. 8.13 and 8.14) – most secure method.
2. Ligation of the cystic duct without rinsing the gall bladder and/or cholecystectomy is the second method of gallbladder treatment during organ procurement. When ligating the cystic duct, you have to be 100% certain that you are not accidentally ligating the duct together with one of the hepatic arteries.
3. Cholecystectomy can be performed at any time during organ procurement, during back-table or even after liver reperfusion.

ATTENTION!
- All manipulations of liver hilum could be very dangerous for the procured liver and the recipient. Cholecystectomy must be safe without damaging the liver hilum structures, especially the arterial vascularisation.

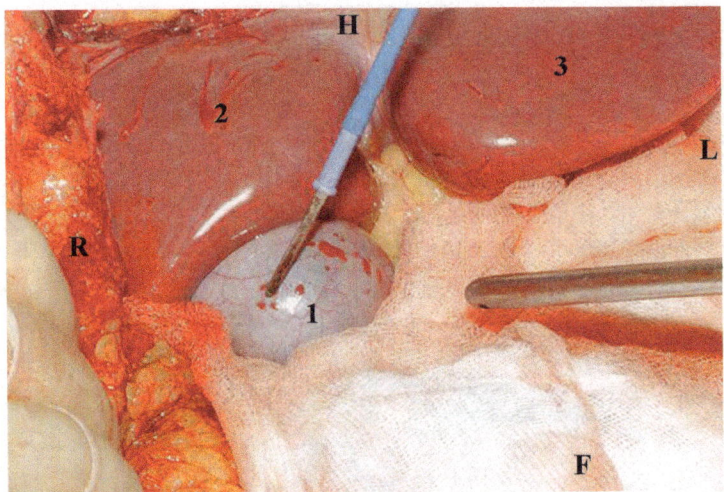

Fig. 8.11 1 – Gallbladder, 2 – Right liver lobe, 3 – Left liver lobe, *H – head, F – feet, R – right, L – left*

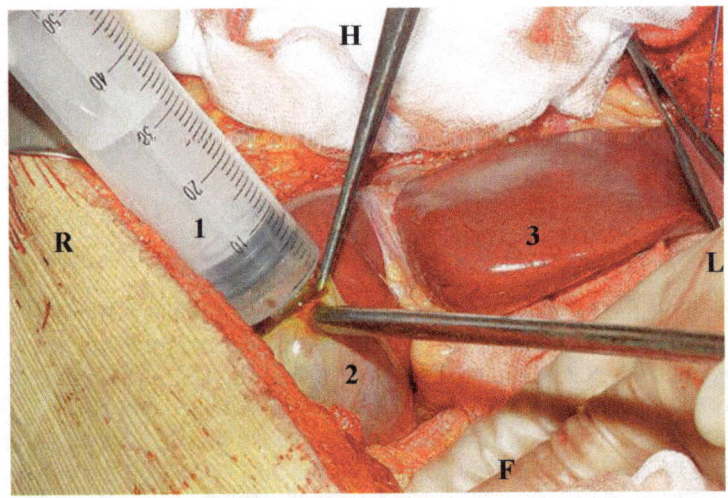

Fig. 8.12 1 – Syringe with warm sterile Ringer or 0.9% NaCl solution, 2 – Opened gallbladder, 3 – Left liver lobe, *H – head, F – feet, R – right, L – left*

8.3 The Gallbladder

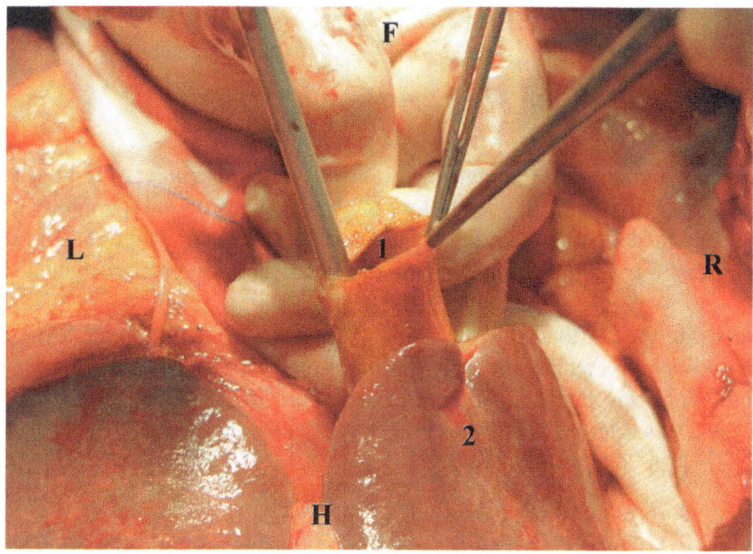

Fig. 8.13 Properly flushed gallbladder. 1 – Cleaned gallbladder, 2 – Right liver lobe, *H – head, F – feet, R – right, L – left*

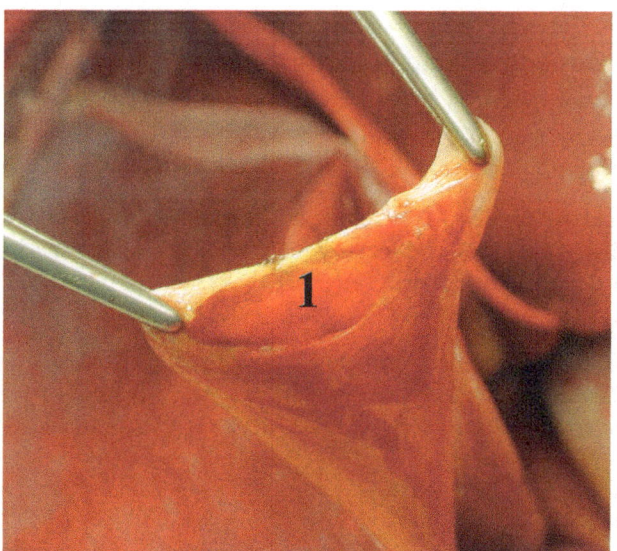

Fig. 8.14 1 – Efficiently flushed, means a properly cleaned gallbladder

8.4 Right Aberrant Hepatic Artery

8.4.1 Anatomy of the Aberrant Hepatic Artery

1. The most frequent type of right aberrant hepatic artery enters the liver on the back side of the pancreas head close to the pancreas capsule; sometimes it is very easy to dissect it from the pancreas without capsule damage. If possible, this artery has to be retrieved with the small cuff or patch from the SMA (1–5).
2. A very rare type of the right aberrant hepatic artery comes from the SMA to the liver through the pancreatic parenchyma. To make the liver and the pancreas suitable for transplantation (after cold perfusion during liver and pancreas splitting), cut this artery at the level of the pancreas parenchyma (1–5).

ATTENTION!
- Only a similar diameter of the right aberrant hepatic artery and the gastroduodenal artery will enable you to make a safe and comfortable anastomosis between them.
- If the arterial anatomy of the liver is unclear, discuss the problem with both recipient transplant surgeons.

8.5 Gastroduodenal and Hepatic Artery Dissection

8.5.1 Surgical Steps

1. Identify and dissect 0.5–1.0 cm of the gastroduodenal and the common hepatic artery (Figs. 8.15–8.17), and localize the anterior side of proper hepatic artery in the hepatoduodenal ligament (Fig. 8.18).

ATTENTION!
- Be alert for an early branching of the common hepatic artery for example low in the space behind pancreas head (own experience).
- To avoid injury, perform a very gentle dissection with very small steps and small angulated vascular clamp.
- Use magnification glasses to avoid pancreas damage and/or spasm of one of the arteries.
- Always look for the right aberrant or right common hepatic artery *Location*: right or posterior side of the portal vein, behind or between CBD and the portal vein.

8.5 Gastroduodenal and Hepatic Artery Dissection

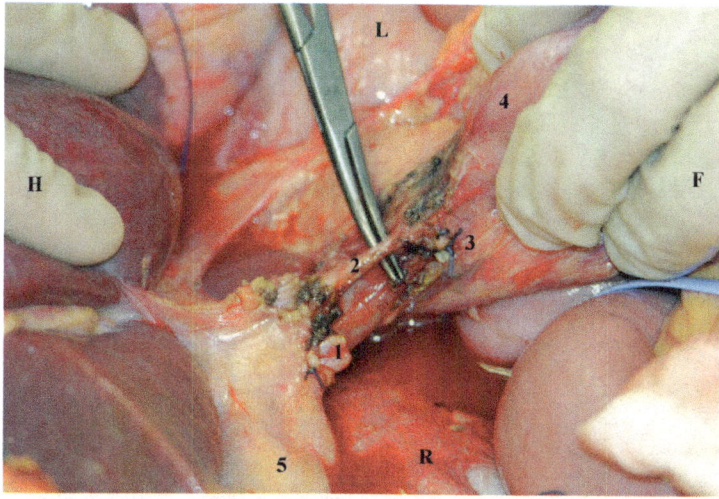

Fig. 8.15 Hepatoduodenal ligament – landmarks. 1 – Cut CBD, 2 – Gastroduodenal artery, 3 – Ligated distal CBD, 4 – Duodenum, 5 – Gallbladder, *H – head, F – feet, R – right, L – left*

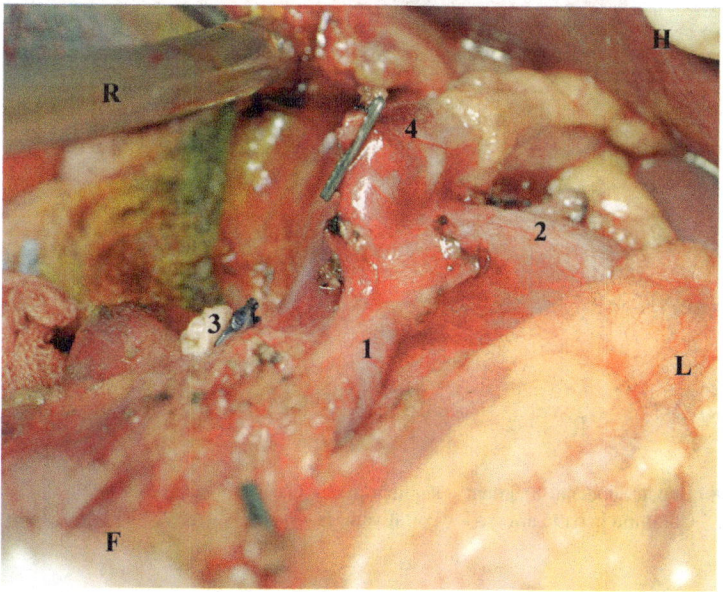

Fig. 8.16 Hepatoduodenal ligament – landmarks. 1 – Gastroduodenal artery, 2 – Common hepatic artery, 3 – Ligated CBD, *H – head, F – feet, R – right, L – left*

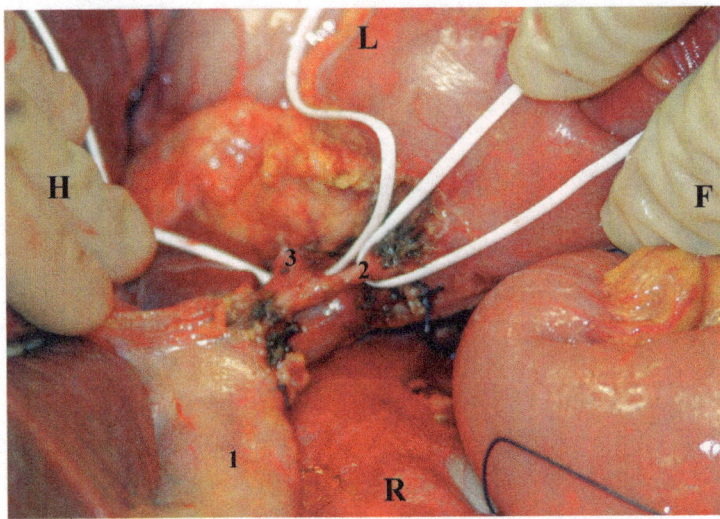

Fig. 8.17 Hepatoduodenal ligament – landmarks. 1 – Gallbladder, 2 – Gastroduodenal artery, 3 – Common hepatic artery, *H – head, F – feet, R – right, L – left*

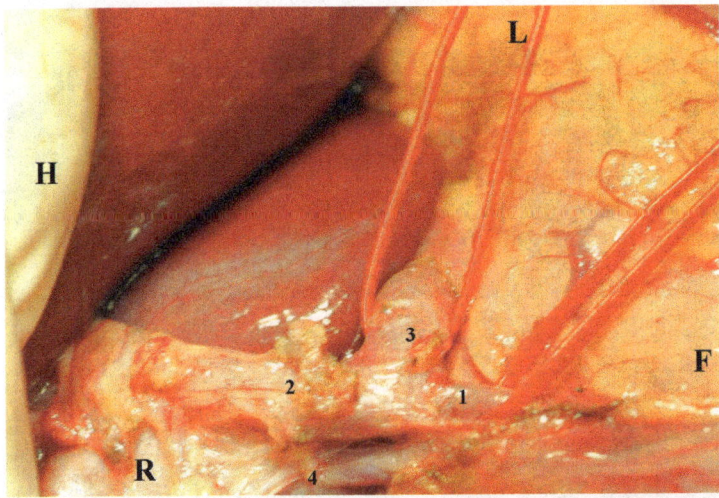

Fig. 8.18 Hepatoduodenal ligament – landmarks. 1 – Gastroduodenal artery, 2 – Proper hepatic artery, 3 – Common hepatic artery, 4 – Portal vein, *H – head, F – feet, R – right, L – left*

8.6 Portal Vein – Dissection

8.6.1 Surgical Steps

1. Free posterior side 1, 5–2 cm of the portal vein begin 0.5 cm above the pancreas parenchyma (Fig. 8.19).

8.6 Literature

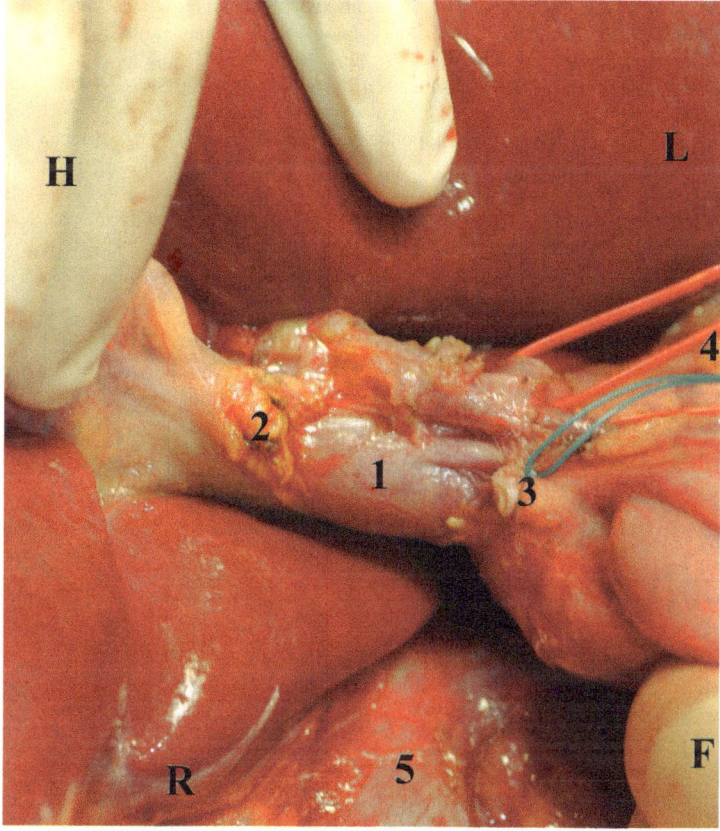

Fig. 8.19 Hepatoduodenal ligament – landmarks. 1 – Portal vein, 2 – Cut proximal CBD, 3 – Ligated distal CBD, 4 – Pancreas, 5 – IVC, *H – head, F – feet, R – right, L – left*

ATTENTION!
If the small bowel is not procured but the rest of the abdominal organs are, go on to Chapter 10.

Literature

1. Skandalakis JE, Branum GD, Colborn GL, Mirilas PS, Weidman TA, Skandalakis LJ, Kingsnorth AN, Zora O (2004) Liver. In Skandalakis PN, Weidman TA, Foster RS Jr, Kingsnorth AN, Skandalakis LJ, Skandalakis PN, Mirilas PS (eds.) Skandalakis Surgical Anatomy. The Embryologic and Anatomic Basis of Modern Surgery, vol. II, Paschalidis Medical Publications, Athens, 1005–1092
2. Skandalakis JE, Branum GD, Colborn GL, Weidman TA, Skandalakis PN, Skandalakis LJ, Zoras O (2004) Extrahepatc biliary tract and gallbladder. In Skandalakis JE, Weidman TA,

Foster Jr RS, Kingsnorth AN, Skandalakis LJ, Skandalakis PN, Mirilas PS (eds.) Skandalakis'Surgical Anatomy. The Embryologic and Anatomic Basis of Modern Surgery, vol. II, Paschalidis Medical Publications, Athens, 1093–1150
3. Van Damme JP, Bonte J (1990) Vascular Anatomy in Abdominal Surgery, Thieme Medical, New York
4. Hesse UJ, Troisi R, Maene L, de Hemptine B, Lameire N (2000) Arterial reconstruction in hepatic and pancreatic allograft transplantation following multi-organ procurement, Transplantation Proceeding: 32: 109–110
5. Mukarami G, Hirata K, Takamuro T, et al (1999) A vascular anatomy of the pancreaticoduodenal region: a review, Journal of Hepatobiliary Pancreatic Surgery: 1: 55–68

Chapter 9
Small Bowel

Abstract Background: Small bowel procurement demands both experience and surgical skill from the surgeon. There are few regional teams in Europe, which are sufficiently experienced in small bowel dissection and procurement. The small bowel, in most cases, is retrieved by the recipient centre team experienced in the field of small bowel retrieval and transplantation. There are a number of different techniques concerning preparation of the intestinal graft, vascular pedicle dissection and finally bowel retrieval. Based on literature, the surgical technique of small bowel dissection is described gradually in this chapter so that it can be easily understood and performed by experienced surgeons.

Conclusion: A well-trained regional team can successfully manage most multi-organ procurements including liver, pancreas, and seldom intestine, from the same donor.

Keywords Small bowel, Small bowel procurement

9.1 Introduction

Improved outcomes in isolated intestinal and multivisceral transplantations have generated a small increase in the demand for multivisceral and isolated small bowel abdominal organ procurement (1).

The small bowel is not procured in most cases of the abdominal multi-organ procurement, because of the small demand, weight mismatch or poor donor condition (1).

The procurement techniques are different and depend on the demands of the recipient (2–7). This chapter describes isolated intestinal procurement without colon, with complete dissection and organ separation in situ according to the technique of Dumont-UCLA Transplant Centre described by Yersis (1). Generally, preparation of the donor before procurement includes selective intestinal decontamination using parenteral and intravenous antibiotics at the time of surgery. An isolated small bowel could be procured with or without the colon and also transplanted in the same way (1–7). Multivisceral or isolated small bowel procurement is one of the more difficult and complicated surgical procedures, which, in most cases, in Europe, are performed by the surgeons from the recipient centre and only seldom by the regional procurement team (4).

9.2 Small Bowel Dissection

9.2.1 Surgical Steps

1. Split with GIA – 55 stapling device the gastrocolic ligament from the pylorus up to the splenic flexure of the colon.
2. Dissect and encircle the pylorus, with a tape.
3. Separate and close the small bowel approximately 2–3 cm below the ligament of Treitz with a GIA – 55 stapling device.

ATTENTION!
- The duodenum is preserved for procurement of the pancreas for transplantation into another patient.

4. With a GIA – 55 stapling device divide the terminal ileum close to the ileocecal valve
5. Continue dissection laterally and distally along the mesocolon outside of the ileocolic superior mesenteric arcade containing the cecal and appendicular vessels.
6. Divide the right, transverse mesocolon and carry the dissection beyond the splenic flexure to completely liberate the colon from the small bowel.
7. Place colon outside the abdomen and go to the vascular pedicles of the small bowel.
8. Gently free and separate the SMA and SMV 2–3 cm below to the uncinate process of the pancreas.
9. Ligate and cut the small branches of the SMA and SMV close to the jejunal wall of the first jejunum loop.
10. Ligate the small pancreatic veins, joining the right part of the SMV.

ATTENTION!
- During dissection avoid the following:
- Unnecessary bleeding
- Pancreas haematoma and iatrogenic injury
- Mesenteric vessels or pancreaticoduodenal arcade damage
- Traction or torsion of the superior mesenteric vessels

Literature

1. Yersiz H, Renz JF, Hisatake GM, Gordon S, Saggi BH et al (2003) Multivisceral and isolated intestinal procurement techniques, Liver Transplantation 9(8): 881–886
2. Jan D, Renz JF (2005) Donor selection and procurement of multivisceral and isolated intestinal allografts, Current Opinion in Organ Transplantation 10: 136–147
3. Di Benedetto F, Quintini C, Lauro A, Masetti M, Cautero N, De Ruvo N, Sassi S, Uso TD, di Francesco F, Romano A, Valle RD, Boggi U, Risaliti A, Ramaccisto G, Pinna AD (2004) Outcome of isolated small bowel and pancreas transplants retrieved from multiorgan donor: the in vivo technique, Transplantation Proceedings 36: 437–438
4. Signori S, Boggi U, Vistoli M, Chiaro MD, Piertrabissa A, Costa T, Bartolo TV, Coletti L, Gemmo F, Croce C, Morelii L, Mosca F (2004) Regional procurement team for abdominal organs, Transplantation Proceedings 36: 435–436
5. Abu-Elmagd K, Fung J, Bueno J, Martin D, Madariaga JR, Mazariegos G, Bond G, Molmenti E, Corry RJ, Starzl TE, Reyes J (2000) Logistics and technique for procurement of intestinal, pancreatic, and hepatic grafts from the same donor, Annals of Surgery 232: 680–687
6. Goulet O, Auber F, Fourcade L, Sarnacki S, Jan D, Columb V, Cézard JP, Aigrain Y, Ricour C, Révillon Y (2002) Intestinal transplantation including the colon in children, Transplantation Proceedings 34: 1885–1886
7. Boggi U, Vistoli F, Del ChiaroM et al (2004) A simplified technique for the en bloc procurement of abdominal organs that is suitable for pancreas and small-bowel transplantation, Surgery 1(35): 629–641

Chapter 10
Thorax Procurement Team(s)

Abstract Background: A tense or competitive atmosphere in the operating room and unprofessional communication skills between members of the thorax and abdominal organ retrieval teams may lead to donor instability, inadequate organ preservation or surgical injury.

During organ procurement, thorax and abdominal teams, which are involved in the organ procurement, have to communicate adequately about the various steps of operation technique, the thoracic organs that have been accepted for transplantation and the time of use of medication with side effects that could be detrimental for the abdominal organs. This applies to the surgical teams, the scrub nurses, the anaesthesia team as well as the transplant coordinators.

Conclusion: If you want to feel content and respected, try to communicate properly.

Co-operation and understanding especially between thorax and abdominal surgeons, during multiorgan procurement – could have a huge influence on the operating room personnel and also on the quality of the procured organs.

Keywords Abdominal organ protection, Thorax procurement team, Thoracic organs dissection, Agreement, Heparinization, Communication skills

10.1 Abdominal Organ Protection

10.1.1 Tip

1. Before the thorax team(s) starts to operate, protect all abdominal organs with 2–3 large, wet gauzes (Fig. 10.1).

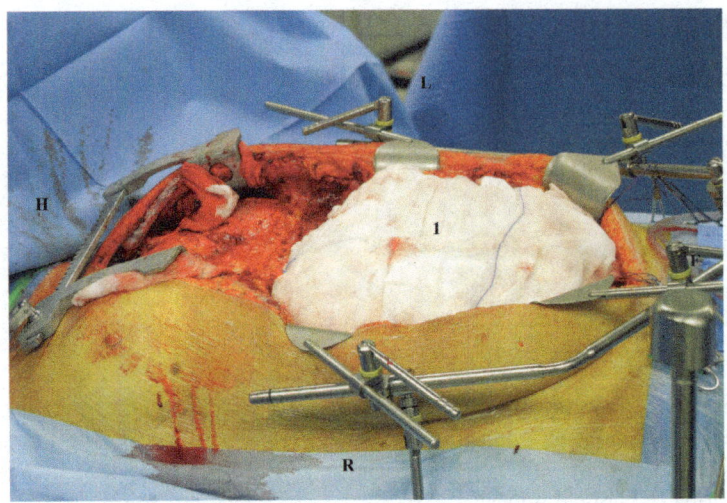

Fig. 10.1 1 – Abdominal organs covered with large, wet gauzes, *H – head, F – feet, R – right, L – left*

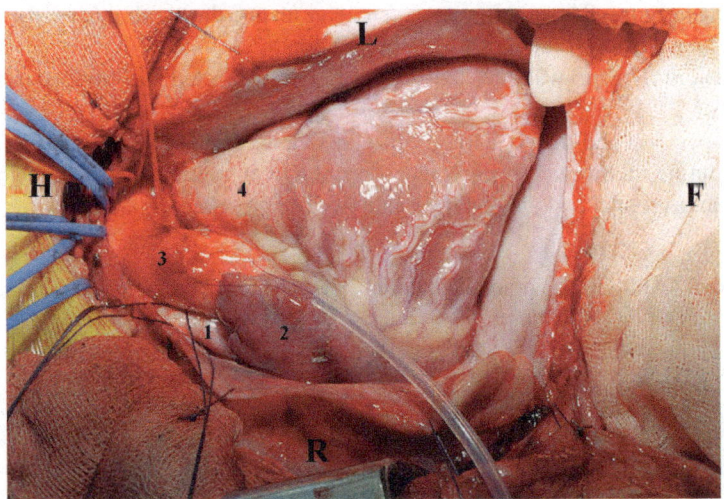

Fig. 10.2 Opened pericardial sack. 1 – Superior vena cava, 2 – Right atrium, 3 – Pulmonary artery, 4 – Aorta, *H – head, F – feet, R – right, L – left*

10.1 Abdominal Organ Protection

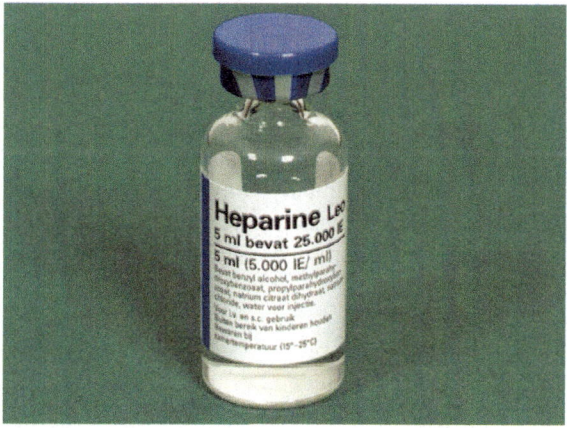

Fig. 10.3 Bottle with heparin (5,000 U heparin mL^{-1})

10.1.2 Dissection of the Thoracic Organs in Sequence

1. Opening of the pericardial sack (Fig. 10.2)
2. Dissection and mobilisation of the thoracic aorta, superior, inferior vena cava, main pulmonary artery and trachea (Fig. 10.3)

ATTENTION!
- Allow the thorax team(s) to dissect the thoracic organs
- Sometimes the distance between the scrub nurse and the thorax team is too big; that is why the abdominal cavity surface is often the best place for collecting surgical instruments
- Try keeping surgical instruments firmly in your hands and avoid dropping them as they could damage the abdominal organs.

10.1.3 An Arrangement with the Thorax Procurement Team(s) About the Following

1. Time and doses of donor heparinization in most of cases: (300–500 U heparin kg^{-1} per donor body weight or 25,000–30,000 U heparin i.v.) – *full heparinization* of the donor (Fig. 10.3)
2. Timing of the major vessel cannulation and start of organ perfusion
3. Use of unusual medication and their effects and side effects before organ perfusion (e.g. Prostaglandin E1)

ATTENTION!
- Remember that prolonged low blood pressure has a side effect. Poor organ perfusion can cause irreversible organ damage and limited organ function after transplantation.
- Heparin will not start to work sooner than 3 min after intravenous injection – there is nothing to do about it, just simply wait.
- Prostaglandin E1 is given via main pulmonary artery causing pulmonary vessels' vasodilatation, and in consequence protects the lungs and the heart against ischemia-reperfusion injury in consequence better lung perfusion.

Chapter 11
Preparation for Organ Perfusion

Abstract Background: After thoracic and abdominal organ dissection, a preservation solution is chosen and preparation for organ perfusion is started. Cold preservation solution is taken from the transport box or refrigerator and afterwards, the surgeon, together with the transplant coordinator and the scrub nurse, prepares the abdominal aorta perfusion system and also, if necessary, the inferior vena cava (IVC) decompression system. At the same time, the thorax team performs similar preparations. The IVC decompression system is not necessary in every case of multi-organ procurement, because the IVC could be also vented into the thorax.

Conclusion: Preparation for abdominal organ perfusion comprises the following steps: choosing (and if necessary preparation of) the preservation solution, abdominal aorta perfusion system and, if necessary, the IVC decompression system.

Keywords UW, HTK, Celsior, Preservation solution, Aorta perfusion system, IVC decompression system

11.1 Preservation Solution

11.1.1 What Is Your Choice UW Or HTK, Or Celsior Preservation Solution?

1. Before perfusion, choose one of the most popular organ preservation solutions:

   - University of Wisconsin (UW) solution about 75–100 mL kg^{-1} per donor body weight (Fig. 11.1)
   - Custodiol histidine-tryptophan-ketoglutarate (HTK) solution about 150–300 mL kg^{-1} per donor body weight (Fig. 11.1)
   - Celsior – 40–60 mL kg^{-1} per donor body weight

11.1.2 Storage

1. Keep the preservation solution cold until organ perfusion, either in the transport box on ice (Fig. 11.2) or in the refrigerator (Fig. 11.3).
2. Ask the transplant coordinator to get the preservation solution from the transport box or refrigerator at the last moment, before organ perfusion.

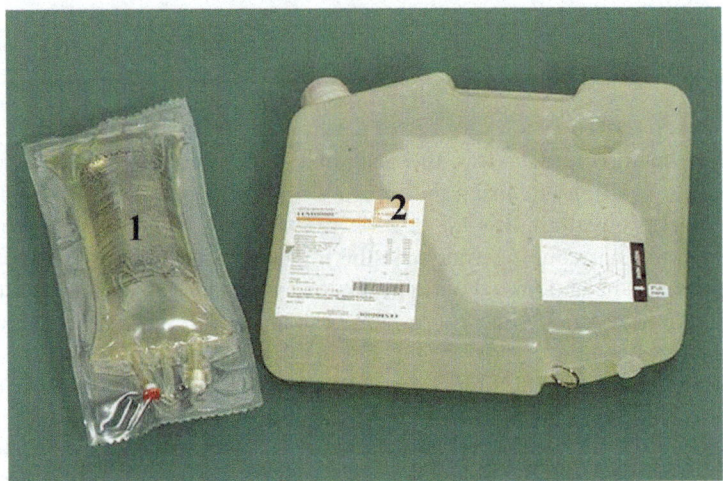

Fig. 11.1 1 – University of Winsconsin (UW) solution, 2 – Custodiol histidine–tryptophan–ketoglutarate (HTK)

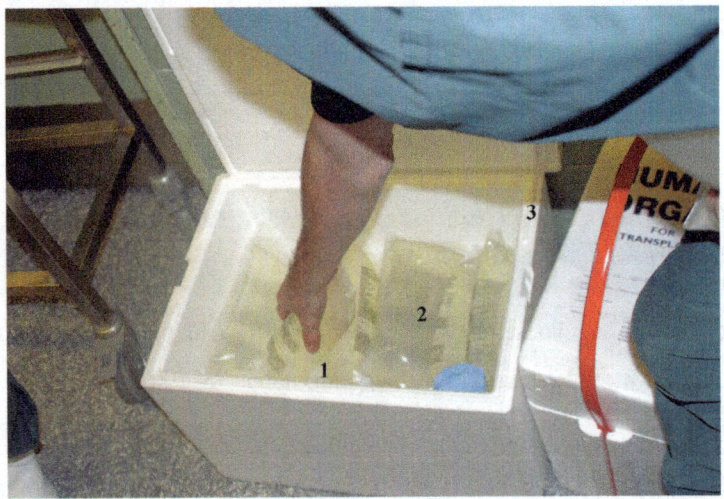

Fig. 11.2 Different cold sterile solutions are kept on ice in the transport box. 1 – Ice, 2 – UW solution, 3 – transport box

11.2 Abdominal Aorta Perfusion System

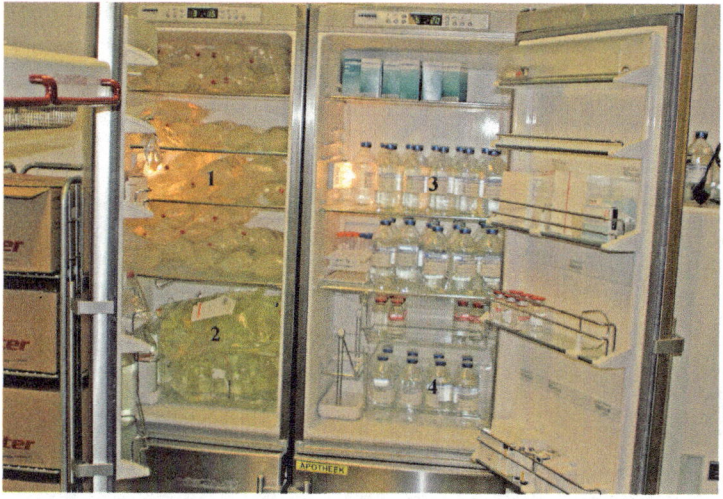

Fig. 11.3 Different cold sterile solutions are kept in the refrigerator. 1 – UW solution and 2 – HTK solution, both in the refrigerator, 3 – Ringer solution, 4 – 0.9% NaCl physiologic solution

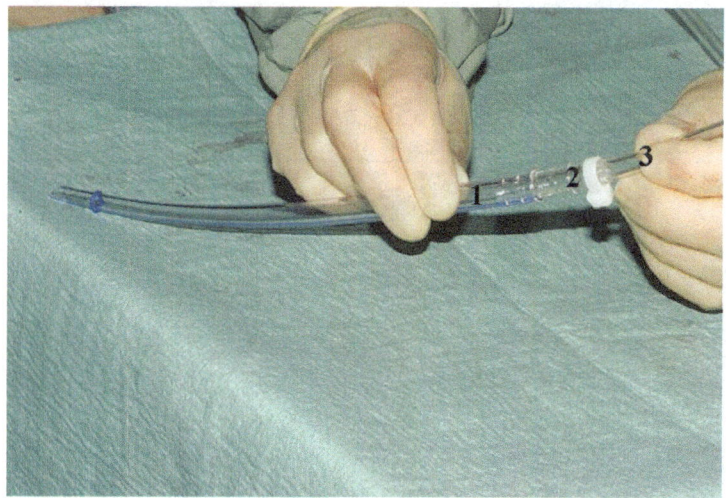

Fig. 11.4 Aorta's perfusion system. 1 – Sterile aortic cannula, 2 – Connection between aortic cannula and rapid perfusion system, 3 – Rapid perfusion system

11.2 Abdominal Aorta Perfusion System

11.2.1 Preparation Technique in Steps

1. Choose the proper diameter of aortic cannula.
2. Connect the end of the sterile rapid perfusion system with the sterile aorta's cannula (Fig. 11.4).

3. Give the other end of the aorta perfusion system to the transplant coordinator and ask him/her for a sterile connection with the container or bags with preservation solution (Fig. 11.5).
4. Fill the rapid perfusion system with cold preservation solution without air and close it with a clamp (Fig. 11.6).

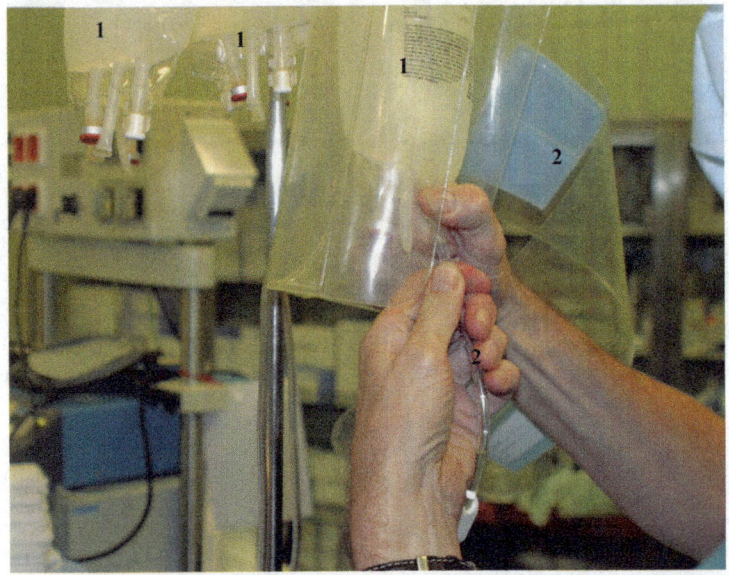

Fig. 11.5 1 – Preservation solution, 2 – Rapid perfusion system

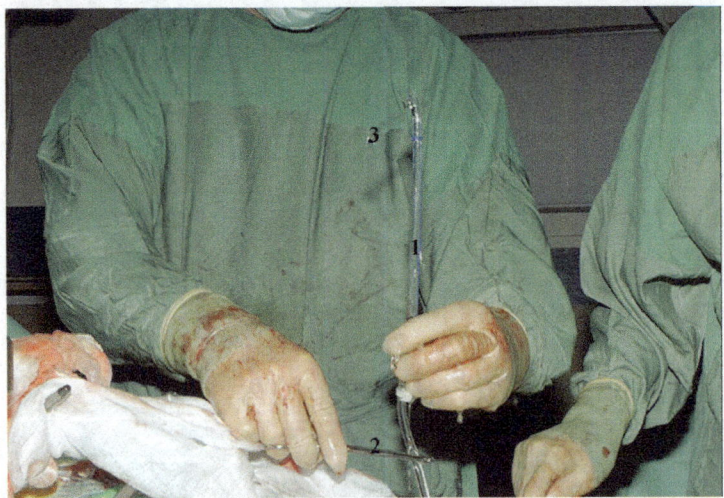

Fig. 11.6 1 – Aortic cannula, 2 – Clamp, 3 – Preservation solution with air coming out from the aortic perfusion cannula

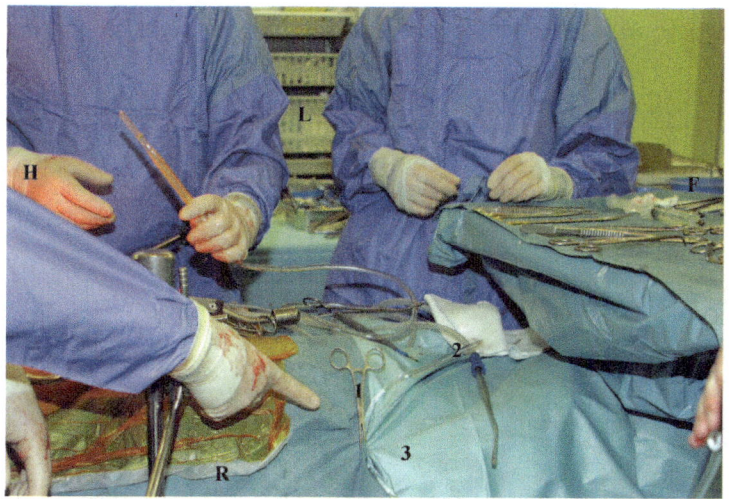

Fig. 11.7 Fix the sterile part of the rapid perfusion system to protect it from falling beyond the sterile operating field. 1 – Clamp, 2 – Sterile part of rapid perfusion system, 3 – Sterile absorbing operating sheet

5. Fix the sterile part of the rapid perfusion system to protect it against falling beyond the sterile operating field (Fig. 11.7).

11.3 Inferior Vena Cava Decompression System

11.3.1 Preparation Technique

1. Prepare the inferior vena cava (IVC) decompression system by connecting the sterile chest tube (22.24;F) with a long silicon tube and close it temporarily with a clamp (Figs. 11.8 and 11.9).

ATTENTION!
- The IVC decompression system is not always necessary; you can also obtain excellent venous decompression by cutting the IVC 2–3 cm above the diaphragm in the direction of the right atrium.
- If the thoracic organs are procured, ask the thoracic surgeon to cut the IVC and decompress the whole system into the thorax cavity.
- Before every HBD organ procurement, I always ask the scrub nurse to have ready all that I need to make my own IVC decompression system, as quickly as possible.

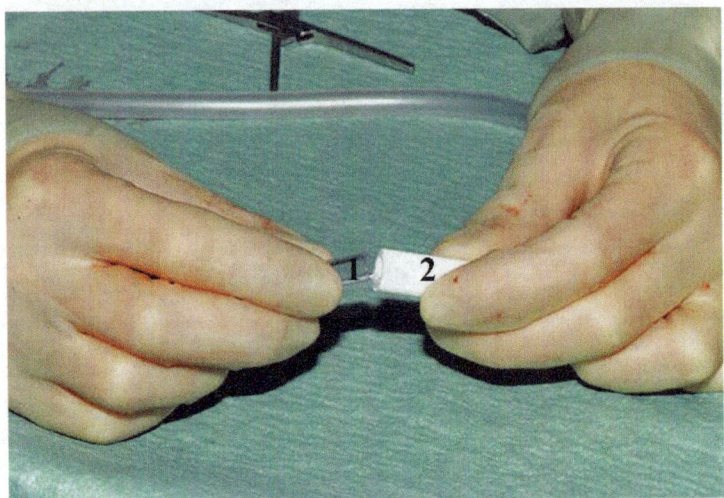

Fig. 11.8 Preparing the IVC decompression system. 1 – Chest tube (22–24°F), 2 – silicon tube

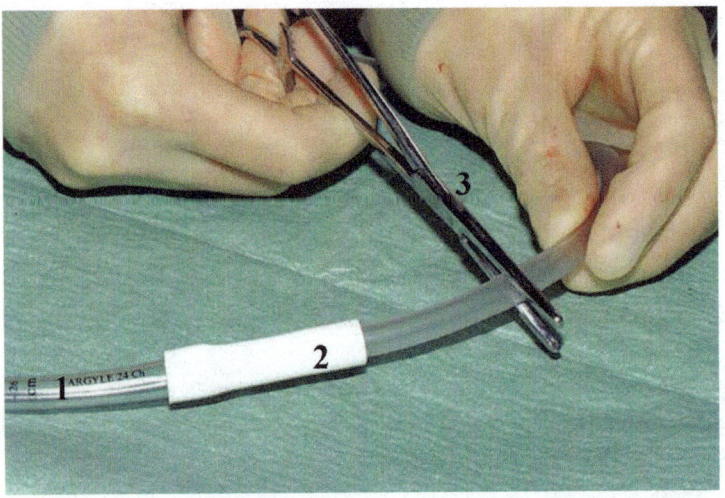

Fig. 11.9 Preparing the IVC decompression system. 1 – Chest tube (22–24°F), 2 – Silicon tube, 3 – Clamp

- If, for any reason, the donor suddenly becomes unstable, before major abdominal vessel cannulation, your *own* decompression system gives you much more chance to start aortic perfusion and decompress the IVC at the same time, and subsequently to rescue the abdominal organs.

Chapter 12
Major Abdominal Vessel Cannulation

Abstract Background: Before abdominal aorta and IVC cannulation, come to an arrangement with the thoracic team about the cannulation. In most cases, where the thoracic organs are procured, the major thoracic vessels are cannulated first followed by the second, abdominal ones. The transplant coordinator(s) and the anaesthetist have to be present in the operating room during major vessel cannulation.
Conclusions: Communicate clearly and on the same level with the procurement teams and with the OR personnel to avoid mistakes during thorax and abdominal major vessel cannulation.

Keywords Abdominal aorta, IVC, Dissection, Preparation for cannulation, Aorta cannulation, IVC cannulation

12.1 Agreement

12.1.1 Communication Skills

1. Before cannulation, come to an understanding with the following:
   - OR personnel
   - Thoracic surgeons (Fig. 12.1)
   - Scrub nurses
   - Anaesthetist
   - Transplant coordinator(s) (Fig. 12.2)

ATTENTION!
- Remember that you are not alone in the operating room; try to communicate adequately with everybody on a professional level.

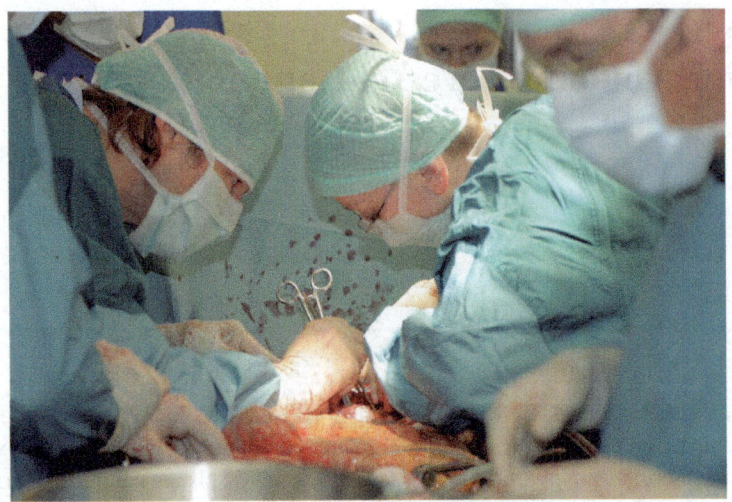

Fig. 12.1 Thoracic surgeons during major thoracic vessel cannulation

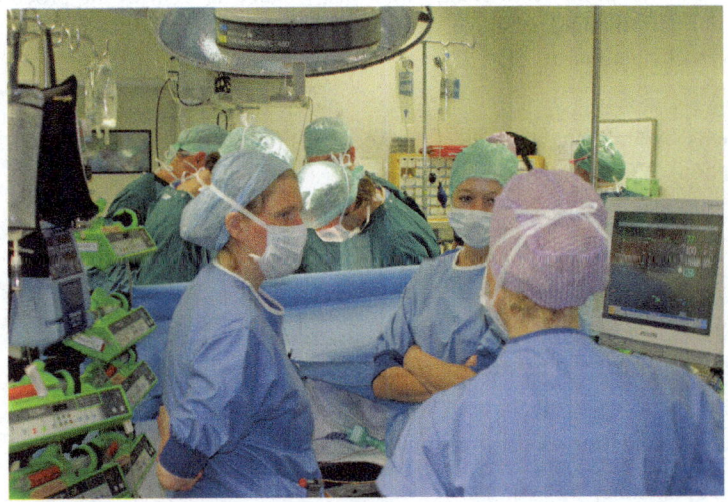

Fig. 12.2 Divide the tasks amongst the OR personnel

12.2 Ligation and Cannulation of the Abdominal Aorta and IVC

12.2.1 Surgical Steps

1. Move the right colon together with the small bowel to the upper part of the abdomen and to the thorax and fix them with an abdominal retractor blade or ask the

thoracic surgeon or your assistant to hold it (Fig. 12.3).
2. Bowel fixating with the retractor blade gives your assistant the opportunity to use both hands and rally help (Fig. 12.4).

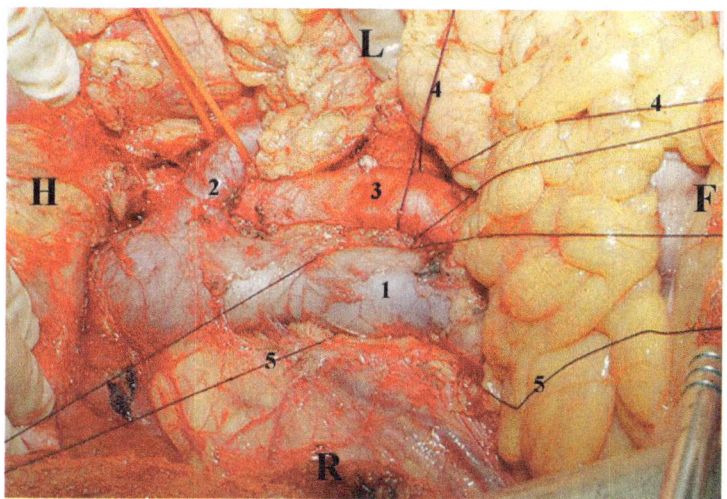

Fig. 12.3 1 – IVC, 2 – Left renal vein, 3 – Abdominal aorta, 4 – Ligature placed around the aorta, 5 – Ligatures placed around the IVC, *H – head, F – feet, R – right, L – left*

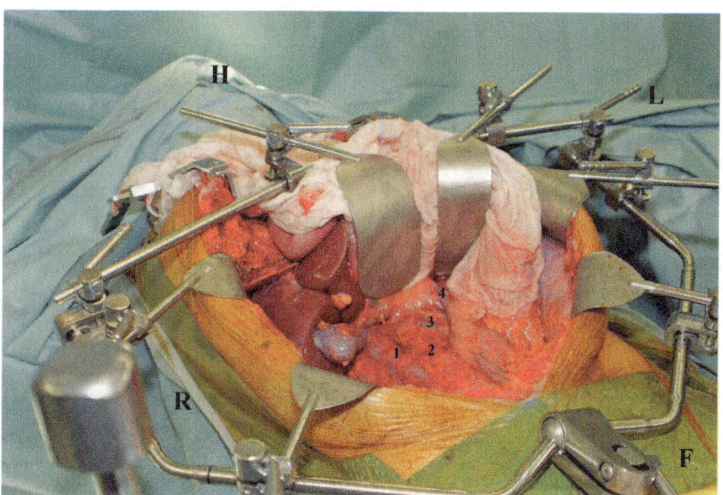

Fig. 12.4 1 – IVC, 2 – Abdominal aorta, 3 – Left renal vein, 4 – IMV, *H – head, F – feet, R – right, L – left*

3. With the first, lowest ligature, ligate the aorta at the level of the bifurcation (Fig. 12.5).
4. Outside the abdominal cavity, fix the ligated ligature with a clamp (Fig. 12.6).

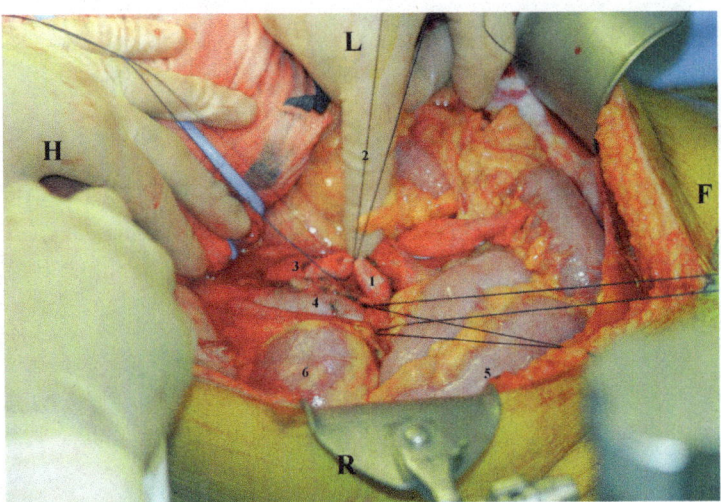

Fig. 12.5 1 – Abdominal aorta at the level of bifurcation, 2 – First lowest ligature placed around the aorta and ligated, 3 – Abdominal aorta above ligation, 4 – IVC, 5 – Sigmoid, 6 – Right kidney, H – head, F – feet, R – right, L – left

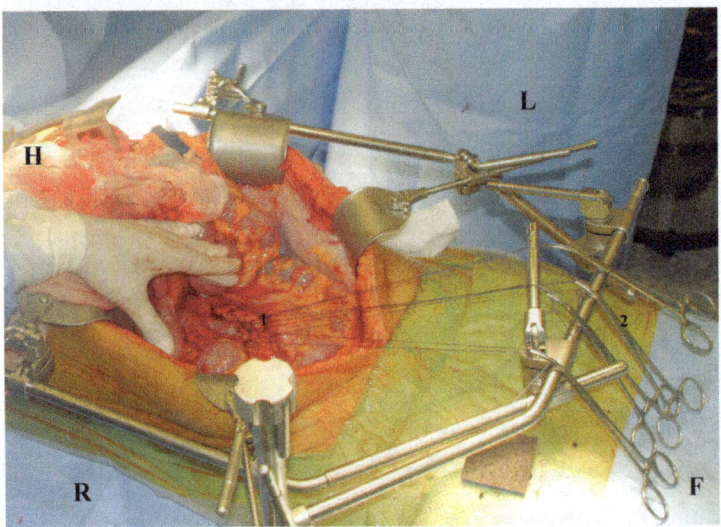

Fig. 12.6 1 – Ligated abdominal aorta, 2 – Ligatures are fixed with the clamps outside abdominal cavity, H – head, F – feet, R – right, L – left

12.2 Ligation and Cannulation of the Abdominal Aorta and IVC

5. Use either the vascular clamp, your fingers or the second upper ligature to close the abdominal aorta below renal arteries.
6. Move the second, upper ligature, 1–2 cm above the place of the planned aorta incision and cut the anterior side of the aorta 1–1.5 cm below the upper ligature (Fig. 12.7).
7. Insert the aortic cannula into the abdominal aorta and secure it with the upper ligature (ligate the aorta on the cannula) and avoid leakage of blood (Fig. 12.8).

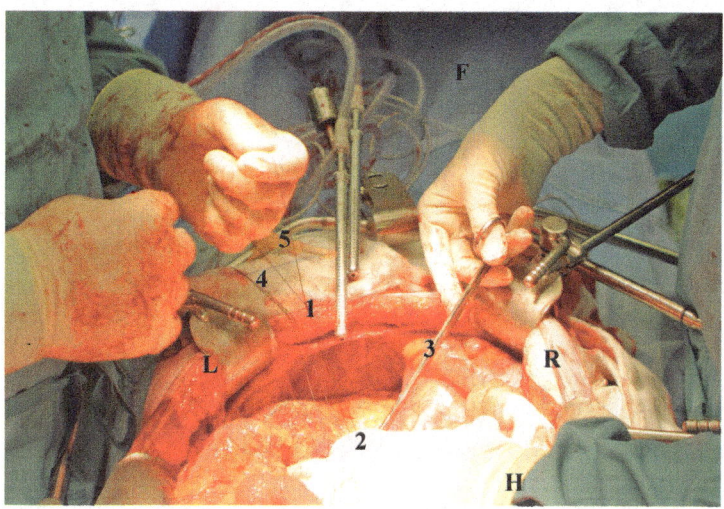

Fig. 12.7 1 – Upper ligature placed around the aorta, 2 – Abdominal aorta is closed with surgeon's fingers, 3 – Scissors, 4 – Lower ligature ligated close to aorta's bifurcation, 5 – Aorta's cannula ready for cannnulation, *H – head, F – feet, R – right, L – left*

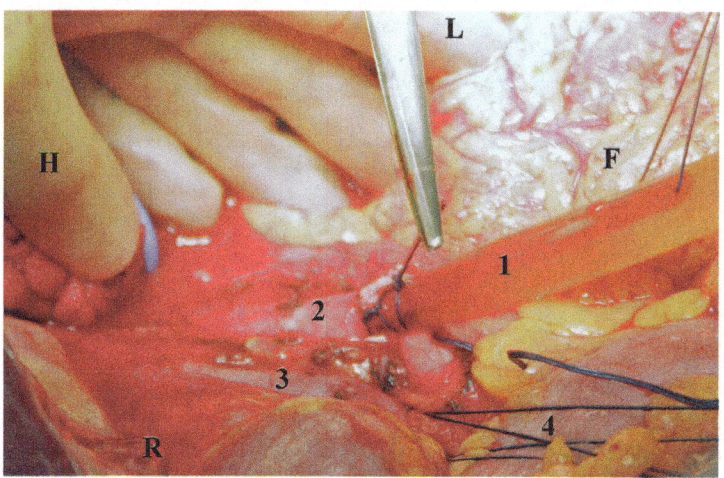

Fig. 12.8 1 – Aortic cannula, 2 – Abdominal aorta, 3 – IVC, 4 – Ligatures placed around the IVC, *H – head, F – feet, R – right, L – left*

8. With the first, lowest ligature, ligate the IVC at the level of their bifurcation and fix the ligature with a clamp outside the abdomen (Fig. 12.9).
9. Use the vascular clamp or your fingers to close the IVC beneath the renal veins.
10. With scissors, cut the anterior side of the IVC about 1–2 cm above the first ligated ligature.

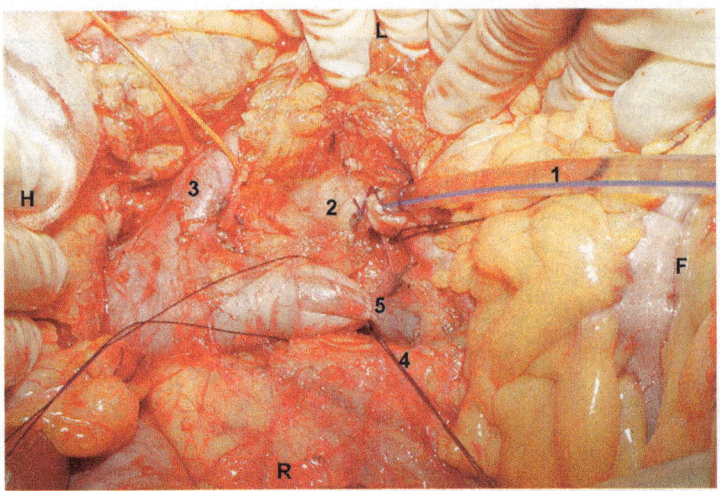

Fig. 12.9 1 – Aortic cannula, 2 – Abdominal aorta, 3 – Left renal vein, 4 – The lowest ligature placed on the IVC, 5 – Ligated IVC close to the bifurcation, *H – head, F – feet, R – right, L – left*

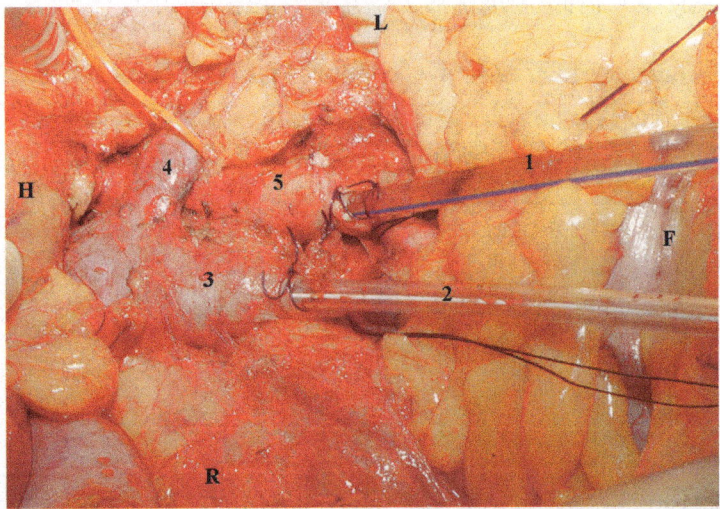

Fig. 12.10 1 – Aortic cannula, 2 – IVC's cannula, 3 – IVC, 4 – Left renal vein, 5 – Abdominal aorta, *H – head, F – feet, R – right, L – left*

12.2 Ligation and Cannulation of the Abdominal Aorta and IVC

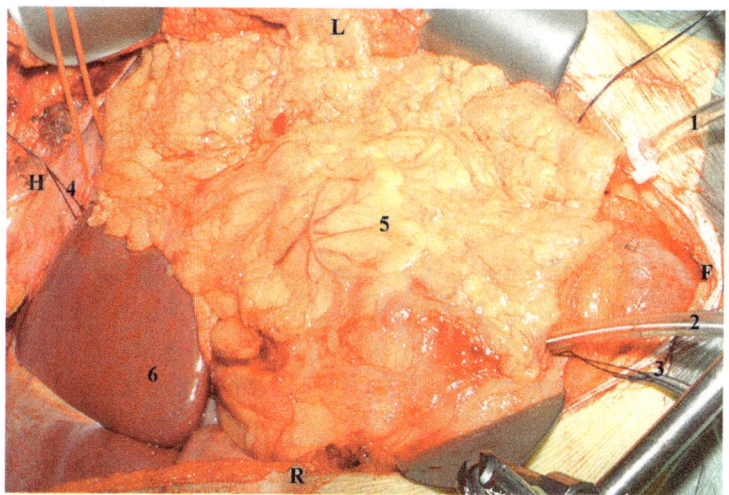

Fig. 12.11 1 – Aortic cannula, 2 – IVC's cannula, 3 – Fixed with clamp ligature, 4 – Ligature around aorta beneath the diaphragm, 5 – Greater omentum, 6 – Left liver lobe, *H – head, F – feet, R – right, L – left*

11. Insert the thorax drain into the IVC and fix it with the second ligature. Avoid leakage of blood.
12. Release the vascular clamps or your fingers from the aorta below the renal arteries and from the IVC and check for leakage along each cannula (Fig. 12.10). In the event of leakage, place a second, new, ligature around the abdominal aorta or IVC or vascular clip where bleeding occurs from the lumbar vessels.
13. Place the colon and the small bowel in the physiologic position back into to the abdomen (Fig. 12.11).

Chapter 13
Cold Perfusion

Abstract Background: Following major vessel cannulation, decide with the thoracic surgeon upon the timing of thoracic and abdominal organ perfusion. The sequence for cold perfusion where multi-organ procurement is envisaged is first the thoracic organs and next the abdominal ones. Both thoracic and abdominal surgeons together with the transplant coordinator must ascertain adequate quality of the thoracic and the abdominal organ perfusion. In case of poor organ perfusion, the aorta cannula should be repositioned or replaced. Continuous adequate topical and internal cooling of abdominal and thoracic organs plays important role during organ procurement and has direct influence on the graft function and patient survival.

Conclusions: Proper internal and external cooling of the thoracic and abdominal organs can have a very important influence on the quality of the organs procured.

Keywords Cold perfusion, Organ perfusion, External cooling, Internal cooling

13.1 Start Thoracic Organ Perfusion

13.1.1 Introduction

First of all start thoracic organ perfusion (Fig. 13.1) while the abdominal organs are still in the physiological position (Fig. 13.2).

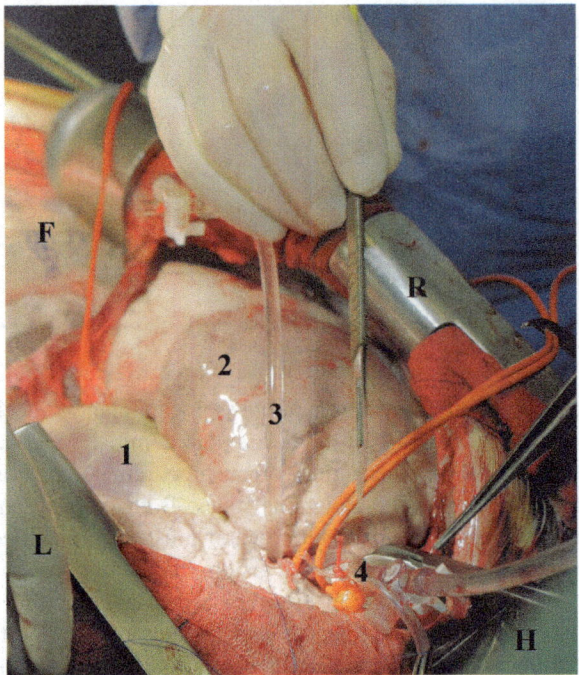

Fig. 13.1 Start thoracic organ perfusion. 1 – Heart, 2 – Right lung, 3 – Aortic cannula, 4 – Pulmonary artery cannula, *H – head, F – feet, R – right, L – left*

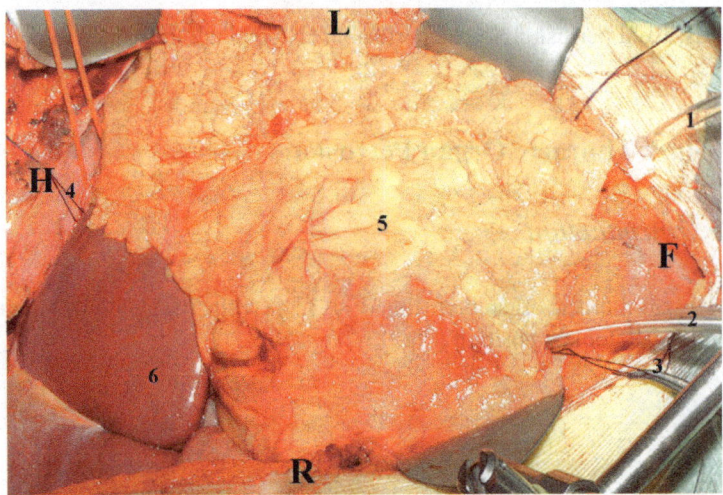

Fig. 13.2 Abdominal organ placed back in the physiological position. 1 – Fixed and closed aortic cannula, 2 – Fixed and closed IVC cannula, 3 – Fixed with clamp IVC ligature, 4 – Ligature placed around aorta beneath the diaphragm, 5 – Greater omentum, 6 – Left liver lobe, *H – head, F – feet, R – right, L – left*

13.2 Start Abdominal Organ Perfusion

13.2.1 Introduction

Immediately after thoracic organ perfusion and abdominal organ perfusion has been started, ask your assistant to gently lift up, protect and move the left liver lobe to the right (Fig. 13.3).

1. If the left liver lobe is well protected, ligate with a thick ligature (Fig. 13.4), or close the abdominal aorta below or above the diaphragm with a clamp (Fig. 13.5).

ATTENTION!
- When the supraceliac aorta is closed with a clamp, there is more risk of left liver vein or left liver lobe parenchyma injury especially when the aorta clamp protrudes above the level of the abdomen and is inhibiting the handling of instruments between the thoracic surgeon and the scrub nurse.
- Sometimes there is too much distance between the thoracic surgeon and the scrub nurse; therefore, they may inadvertently dislodge the abdominal aortic clamp.

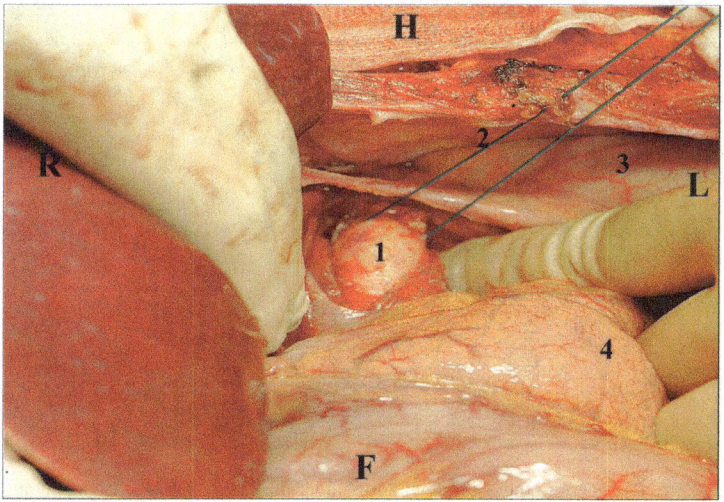

Fig. 13.3 Left liver lobe protected with the hand. 1 – Abdominal aorta below the diaphragm, 2 – Ligature, 3 – Stomach, 4 – Pancreas, *H – head, F – feet, R – right, L – left*

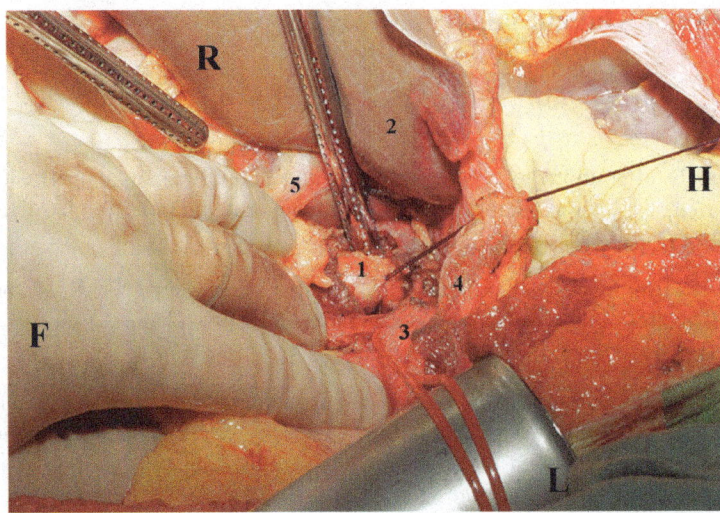

Fig. 13.4 1 – Ligated abdominal aorta beneath the diaphragm, 2 – Left liver lobe, 3 – Oesophagus, 4 – Diaphragm, *H – head, F – feet, R – right, L – left*

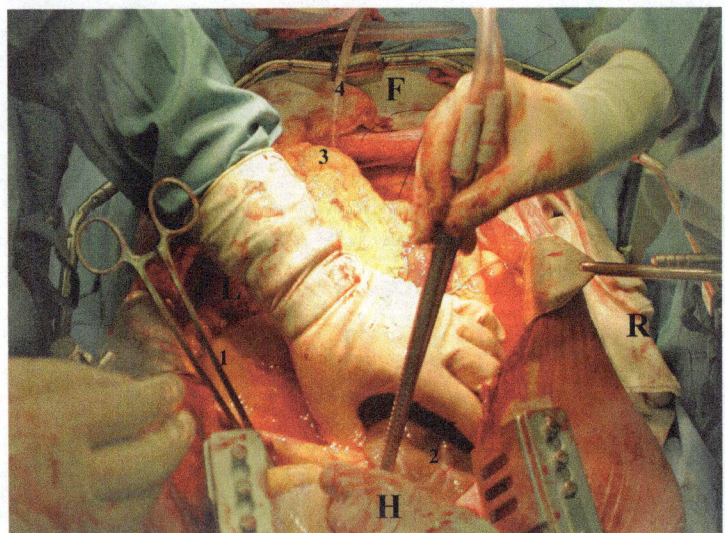

Fig. 13.5 Difficult access to the abdominal aorta under the diaphragm. 1 – Clamped aorta in the left thorax 10 cm above the diaphragm, 2 – Left liver lobe, 3 – Small bowel, *H – head, F – feet, R – right, L – left*

13.2.2 Clamp Removal

1. Remove both clamps from the silicon tubes and start cold abdominal organ perfusion (Fig. 13.6).

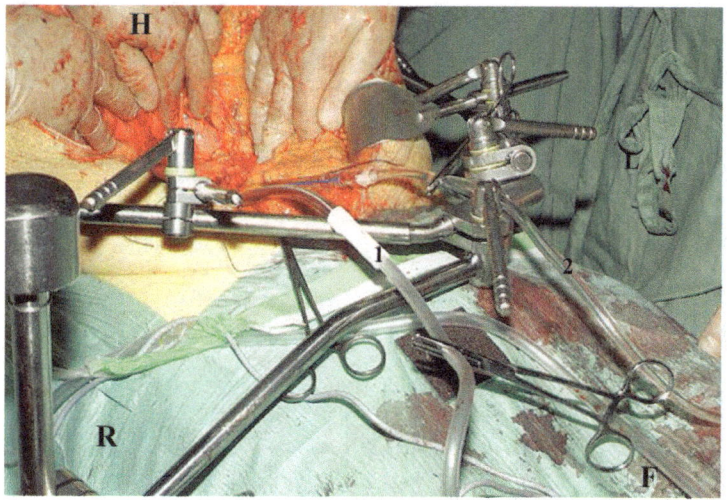

Fig. 13.6 1 – IVC decompression system, 2 – Aortic cannula, *H – head, F – feet, R – right, L – left*

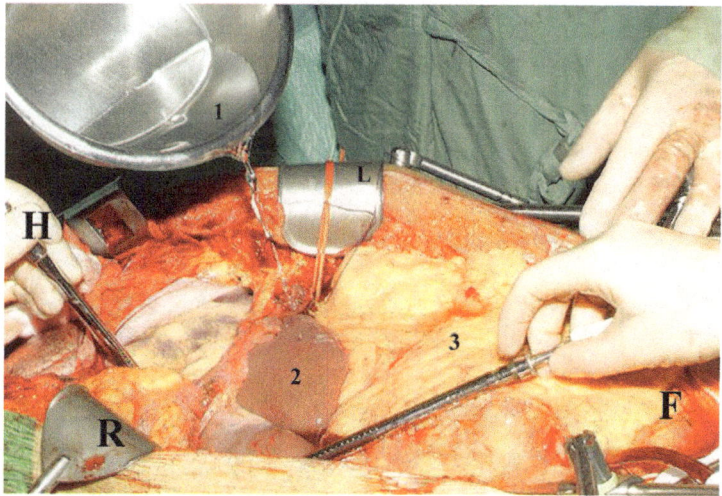

Fig. 13.7 Abdominal external topical cooling. 1 – Cold sterile Ringer solution, 2 – Left liver lobe, 3 – Greater omentum, *H – head, F – feet, R – right, L – left*

13.2.3 Topical Cooling

1. At the same time begin continuous topical (external) abdominal cooling of the thoracic organs. Use cold sterile Ringer lactate or 0.9% NaCl solution (Fig. 13.7) and sterile ice or ice-slush (Fig. 13.8). Replace them regularly.

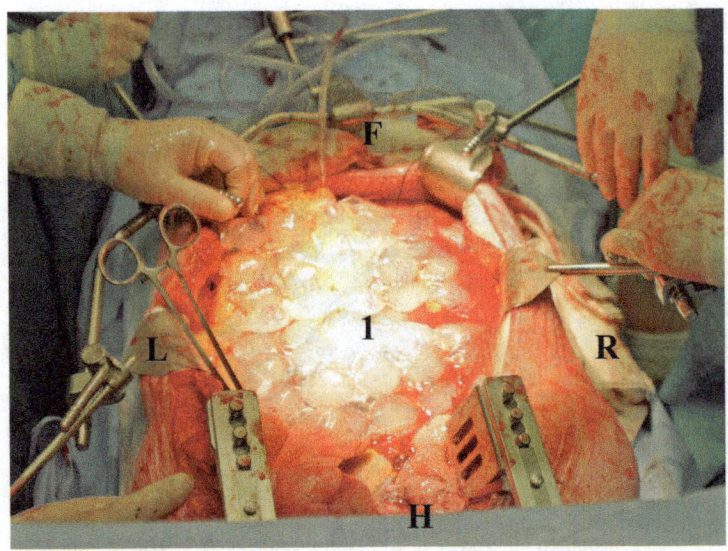

Fig. 13.8 Topical cooling of abdominal organs. 1 – Sterile ice, *H – head, F – feet, R – right, L – left*

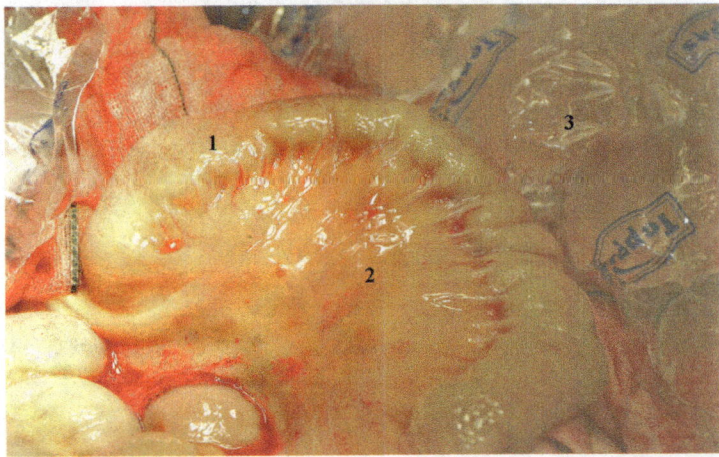

Fig. 13.9 Quality of abdominal organ perfusion. 1 – Small bowel, 2 – Mesentery of the small bowel, 3 – Sterile ice

13.2.4 Check Efficiency of the Abdominal Organ Perfusion System

1. First ask the transplant coordinator about any obstruction to the perfusion system.
2. Observe and ensure that the mesentery of the small bowel is free of blood (Fig. 13.9).

13.2 Start Abdominal Organ Perfusion

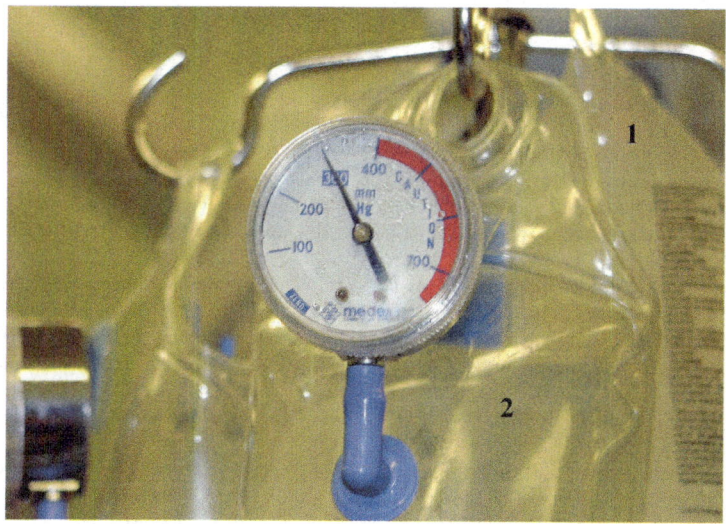

Fig. 13.10 1 – Bag of UW solution, 2 – Preservation solution under the pneumatic pressure of 300 mmHg

3. In case of poor organ perfusion or insufficient decompression, replace or reposition aorta and/or the IVC cannula.
4. Cutting totally the IVC in the abdomen or at the level of the right atrium should be helpful during decompression of the IVC.

ATTENTION!
Most retrieval teams perfuse the abdominal organs at a relatively low pressure of 80–100-cm H_2O (gravity). Some prefer to perfuse the aorta at a higher pressure (150 mmHg). In the Netherlands, we use, in my opinion, one of the highest pressures, namely 300 mmHg.

The reason for this high pneumatic pressure is to simulate the physiological organ perfusion and obtain about 80-mmHg pressure in the abdominal aorta. As mentioned, to achieve this value of pressure, you have to put about 300-mmHg pneumatic pressure on the perfusate bag (Fig. 13.10).

During abdominal organ perfusion, the pressure obtained in the abdominal aorta is close to 80 mmHg and is almost equal to the physiologic perfusion pressure of abdominal organs (1, 2, 3, 4, 5, 6, 7).

The second question is always – what is the best method of abdominal organ perfusion: *single* or *dual* perfusion; single perfusion consists of cannulation and perfusion of only the abdominal aorta or cannulation of the aorta and the portal vein – dual perfusion. On the basis of the literature, my conclusion is that the single cannulation of the aorta is superior to combined aortic and portal vein cannulation. This applies to all the retrieved abdominal organs and is most important when the pancreas or intestine is to be transplanted (7, 8, 9, 10, 11, 12, 13, 14, 15).

Literature

1. Iaria G, Tisone G, Pisani F et al (2001) High-pressure perfusion versus gravity perfusion in liver harvesting: results from a prospective randomized study. Transplant Proc: 33: 957–958
2. Tisone G, Vennarecci G, Baiocchi L et al (1997) Randomized study on in situ liver perfusion techniques: gravity perfusion vs high-pressure perfusion. Transplant Proc: 29: 3460–3462
3. Tisone G, Orlando G, Pisani F et al (1999) Gravity perfusion versus high-pressure perfusion in kidney transplantation: results from a prospective randomized study. Transplant Proc: 31: 3386–3387
4. Komokata T, Nishida S, Ogata S et al (1998) Influence of the flow rate during flushing on porcine multivisceral preservation. In Vivo: 12: 245–251
5. Tokunaga Y, Ozaki N, Wakashiro S et al (1988) Effects of perfusion pressure during flushing on the viability of the procured liver using noninvasive fluorometry. Transplantation: 45: 1031–1035
6. Chui AK, Thompson JF, Lam D et al (1998) Cadaveric liver procurement using aortic perfusion only. Aust N Z J Surg: 68: 275–277
7. Brockman JG, Vaida A, Reddy S, Friend PJ (2006) Retrieval of abdominal organs for transplantation. Br J Surg: 93: 133–146
8. Komokata T, Nishida S, Ogata S et al (1998) Influence of the flow rate during flushing on porcine multivisceral preservation. In Vivo: 12: 245–251
9. Tokunaga Y, Ozaki N, Wakashiro S et al (1988) Effects of perfusion pressure during flushing on the viability of the procured liver using noninvasive fluorometry. Transplantation: 45: 1031–1035
10. Chui AK, Thompson JF, Lam D et al (1998) Cadaveric liver procurement using aortic perfusion only. Aust N Z J Surg: 68: 275–277
11. de Ville de Goyet J, Hausleithner V, Malaise J et al (1994) Liver procurement without in situ portal perfusion. A safe procedure for more flexible multiple organ harvesting. Transplantation: 57: 1328–1332
12. Gabel M, Liden H, Norrby J et al (2001) Early function of liver grafts preserved with or without portal perfusion. Transplant Proc: 33: 2527–2528
13. Colledan M, Doglia M, Fassati LR et al (1998) Liver perfusion in multiorgan harvesting for transplantation. Transplant Proc: 20: 847–848
14. Marino IR, De Luca G, Celli S et al (1998) Comparison of combined portal-arterial versus portal perfusion during liver procurement. Transplant Proc: 20 (Suppl 1): 578–587
15. Filipponi F, Oleggini M, Romagnol P et al (1996) Exclusively aortic cold flushing for liver procurement from haemodynamically stable donors. An experimental study in the pig. Giornale di Chirurgia (G. Chir), Jan-Feb; 17(1–2): 59–63

Chapter 14
Thoracic Organ Procurement

Abstract Background: After external and internal organ cooling and preservation, the first thoracic organs are procured. During lung retrieval, the anaesthetist must be present in the OR. Procured organs are packed according to the international or national rules and put on ice in special transport boxes. To safeguard the organ recipient, at the end of the procedure, even if only one of the organs has been retrieved from the thorax cavity, the abdominal surgeon must inspect the rest of the organ including the thoracic wall for signs of cancer or other risk-increasing complications or disease.

Conclusion: Because of short ischemia time, the thoracic organs have to be well preserved, quickly procured and transplanted as quickly as possible. The abdominal surgeon must inspect the remaining organs (after thorax and abdominal organ procurement) including the thorax wall for signs of cancer.

Keywords Heart procurement, Lungs procurement, Thoracic organ procurement

14.1 Introduction

After external and internal cooling and preservation as described earlier, different combinations of thoracic organs are procured. During lung retrieval, the anaesthetist must be present in the OR to inflate the lungs and to withdraw the endotracheal tube. Thoracic organs are packed according to international or national rules, in three separate sterile bags, which are closed without air and then put on ice in the special transport boxes. The first bag is always filled with a preservation solution, the second with cold saline or Ringer and the third, in most cases, is kept dry. During thoracic organ procurement the short ischemic time plays a very important role. Most cardiac teams require approximately 20–40 min from the onset of cardioplegic infusion to completion of the cardiectomy (1). The heart tolerates cold ischemia poorly, and during retrieval it should be well preserved, quickly procured and transplanted as quickly as possible. To safeguard the organ recipient, after procurement, at the end of the procedure, the abdominal surgeon must inspect the remaining organ or organs in the thoracic cavity for signs of cancer or other risk-increasing complications or disease.

14.1.1 Sequence of Abdominal Organ Procurement

1. The thoracic organs are procured in the following sequence:
   - First the heart (Fig. 14.1). Here, care must be taken to leave enough supra-diaphragmatic IVC for both organs such as the liver and the heart (Figs. 14.2 and 14.3).
   - Then the lungs separately or together (Fig. 14.4).
   - Finally, heart and lungs together (Fig. 14.5).

ATTENTION!
- The abdominal organ cooling has to be continued until the last thoracic organ is procured (Fig. 14.6).

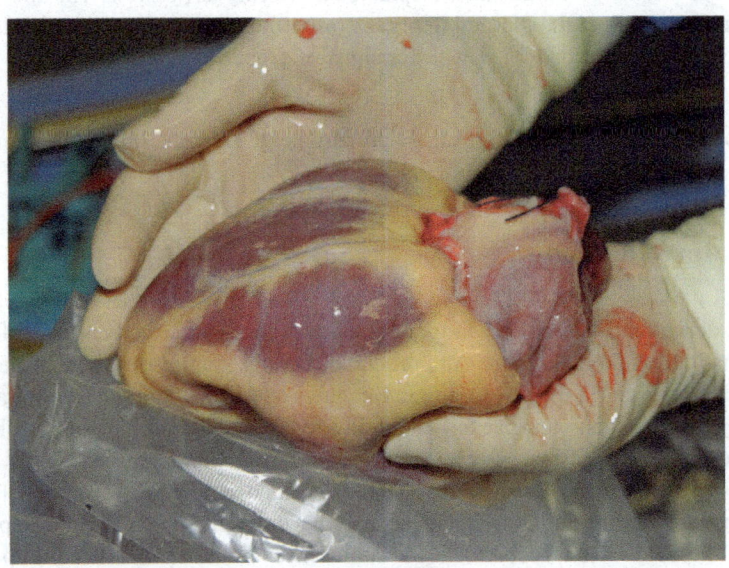

Fig. 14.1 Procured heart before packing

14.1 Introduction

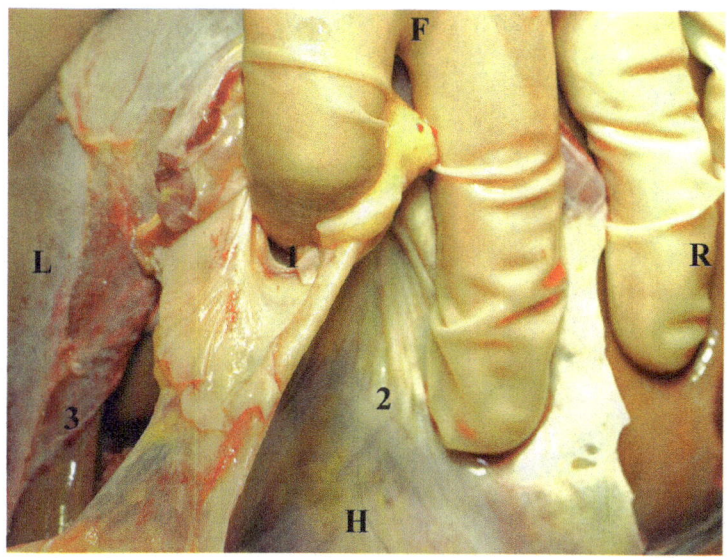

Fig. 14.2 1– Supradiaphragmatic IVC, 2 – Right diaphragm, 3 – Left liver lobe, *H – head, F – feet, R – right, L – left*

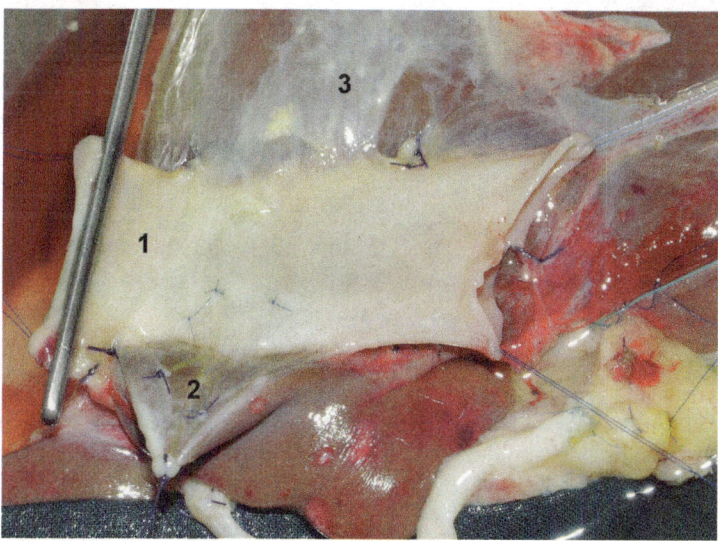

Fig. 14.3 Liver inspection before transplantation – back-table. 1 – Supradiaphragmatic IVC must be long enough to close it before transplantation or anastomose with the IVC of the recipient 2 – Caudate liver lobe, 3 – Right liver lobe

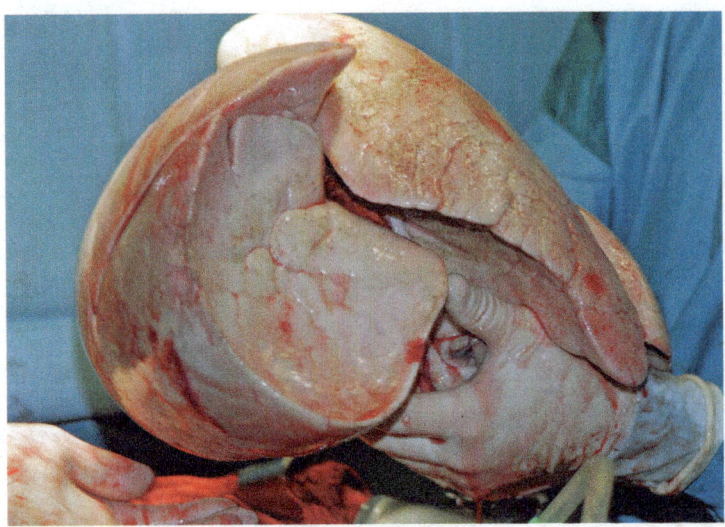

Fig. 14.4 Procured lungs before packing

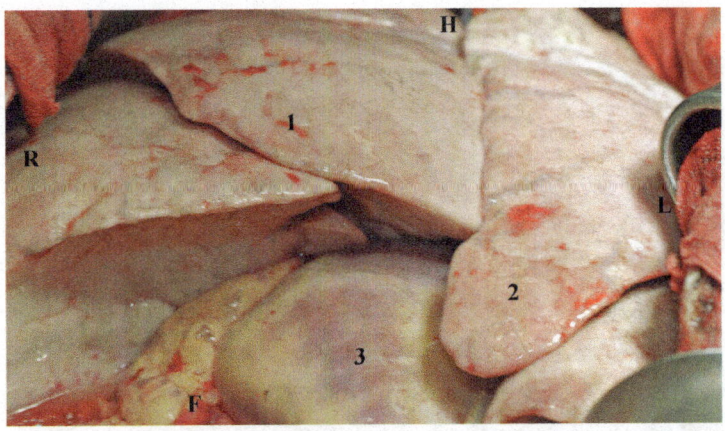

Fig. 14.5 Heart and lungs together after cold perfusion before procurement. 1 – Right lung, 2 – Left lung, 3 – Heart, *H – head, F – feet, R – right, L – left*

- To safeguard the organ recipient, after procurement, at the end of the procedure, the remaining organ or organs in the thoracic cavity must be inspected by the abdominal surgeon for signs of cancer or other risk-increasing complications or disease (Fig. 14.7).

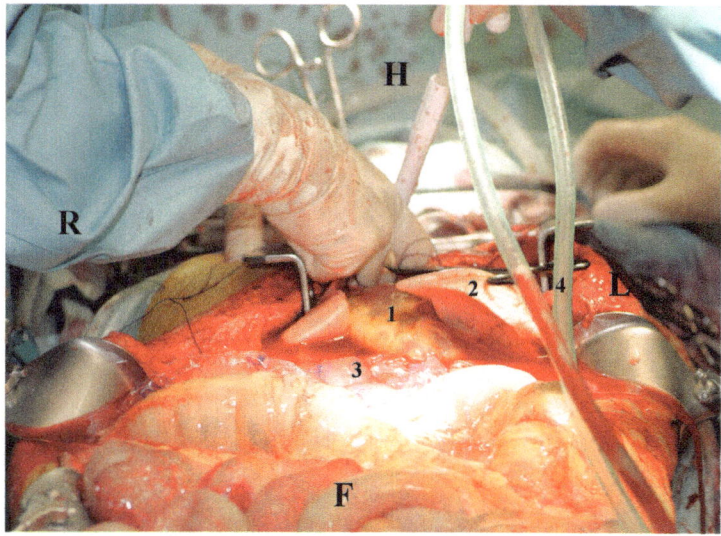

Fig. 14.6 Continuous internal and external cooling of abdominal organs during thoracic organ procurement. 1 – Heart, 2 – Left lung, 3 – Sterile ice with cold sterile solution, 4 – Suction system, H – head, F – feet, R – right, L – left

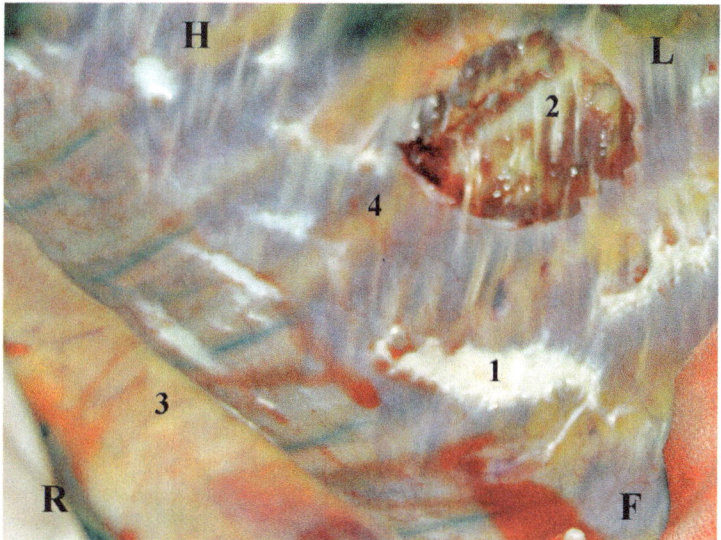

Fig. 14.7 Disease of the thoracic wall found at the end of multi-organ procurement by the abdominal surgeon following heart procurement. 1 – Pathological change, 2 – Thoracic wall biopsy place, 3 – Vertebral column

Literature

1. Florman SS, Starzl TE, Miller ChM (2003) ASC Surgery. http://www.medscape.com/viewarticle/449855

Chapter 15
Sequence of Abdominal Organ Procurement

Abstract Background: Where all organs were accepted and, after inspection, are found to be suitable for transplantation, the following sequence of abdominal organ procurement is recommended: small bowel, pancreas, liver, kidneys. The small bowel is the most sensitive organ for ischemia; therefore, it is retrieved first.

The second organ to be procured from the abdomen is the pancreas followed by the liver or vice versa. Liver and the pancreas could also be retrieved *en block* and split on the back table. In some cases, the pancreas should be offered up for the liver (small donor, very difficult recipient, anatomical abnormality), especially when the risk of arterial damage due to anatomical abnormality or thrombosis is high and the arterial vascularization is uncertain. Finally, the kidney(s) is/are the last organ(s) to be procured. There are many different surgical techniques concerning kidney retrieval with splitting in the abdomen in situ or procurement together followed, if necessary, with splitting on the back table. For many reasons, in most donation procedures, the small bowel is not accepted for procurement and transplantation. In a small number of cases, if the small bowel has been accepted it is procured by the regional procurement team, but more usually by the transplant surgeons from the small bowel recipient centre.

In this chapter, I pay special attention to describe step by step the most frequent occurrence facing the regional procurement surgeon when the small bowel is not procured from the abdominal cavity and the rest of the organs are procured.

Conclusion: A good surgical procurement technique and very good knowledge of human anatomy are the two important things, which allow you proper recognition of the most important vascular abnormalities during organ dissection. These two skills will help you to avoid surgical mistakes, which would otherwise lead to organ damage.

Keywords Pancreas, Small bowel, Liver, Kidneys, Organ procurement, Organ splitting, Vascular splitting, Procurement

15.1 Small Bowel Procurement

If the small bowel (1–7) is not procured but the rest of the abdominal organs are procured, then see Sect. 15.2.

15.1.1 Surgical Steps

1. Before or after cold perfusion, mark with vessel loop the border between Treitz ligament and the jejunum.
2. Divide duodenum from the jejunum at the level of the Treitz ligament. Use a 55-mm gastrointestinal stapling device (GIA).
3. Ligate or cut the dissected mesenteric vessels (SMA and SMV) from the pancreas and the small bowel side.
4. Place the small bowel in a sterile container filled with either ice or cold sterile 0.9% NaCl, Ringer lactate or preservation solution.
5. Pack it according to national or international rules.
6. A good quality *tool-kit* has to be packed according to the same rules as that for retrieved organs.

ATTENTION!
- The small bowel is the first organ to be procured from the abdominal cavity.
- To achieve minimal cold ischemia time, the small bowel could in the most cases be harvested before or after heart and lungs.

If the small bowel was procured, then see Sect. 15.4.

15.2 Pancreas, Liver and Kidneys Procurement Surgical Technique

15.2.1 Introduction

As I have already mentioned in Chap. 9, small bowel procurement demands experience and surgical skills from the surgeon. There are not many regional teams in Europe that are experienced in small bowel procurement. The small bowel, in most cases, is retrieved by the recipient centre team experienced in the field of small bowel retrieval and transplantation. In this section, I first want to describe the most frequent occurrence facing the regional procurement surgeon when the small bowel is not procured from the abdominal cavity and the rest of the organs are. In such a case, the surgeon is confronted with the following situation in the abdominal cavity:

15.2 Pancreas, Liver and Kidneys Procurement Surgical Technique

- No small bowel mesenteric root dissection has been done earlier.
- The level of the pylorus (Fig. 15.1) and Treitz ligament (Fig. 15.2) could be marked with a vessel loop before or after cold perfusion.

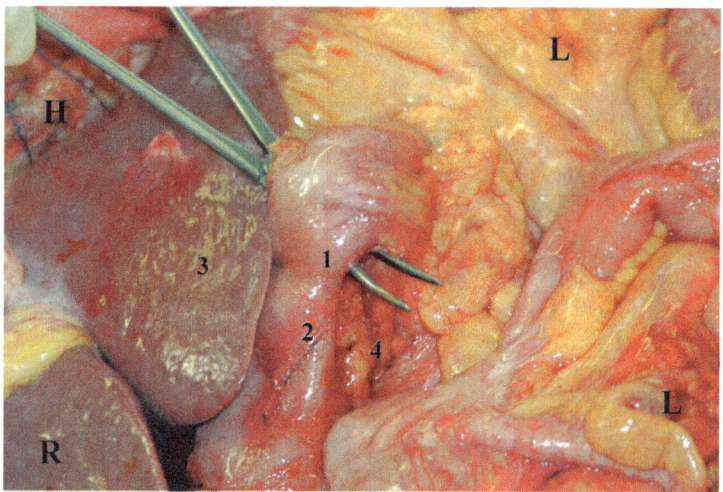

Fig. 15.1 Before cold perfusion, the level of the pylorus will be marked with a vessel loop. 1 – Pylorus, 2 – Duodenum, 3 – Left liver lobe, 4 – Pancreas, *H – head, F – feet, R – right, L – left*

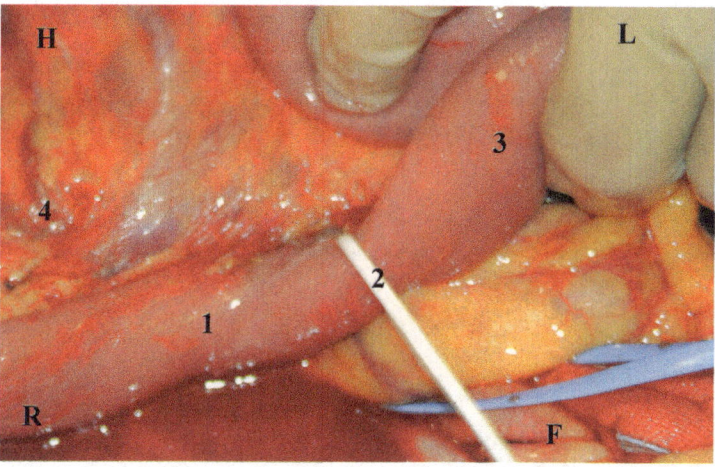

Fig. 15.2 Level of the Treitz ligament is marked with a vessel loop. 1 – Duodenum (ascending part), 2 – Vessel loop, 3 – Jejunum, 4 – Pancreas head, *H – head, F – feet, R – right, L – left*

15.2.2 Sterilizing Duodenum Content

1. Divide the duodenum from the jejunum at the level of Treitz ligament. Use a 55-mm GIA (Figs. 15.3 and 15.4).
2. Replace the gastric tube from the stomach to the duodenum (Figs. 15.5 and 15.6).

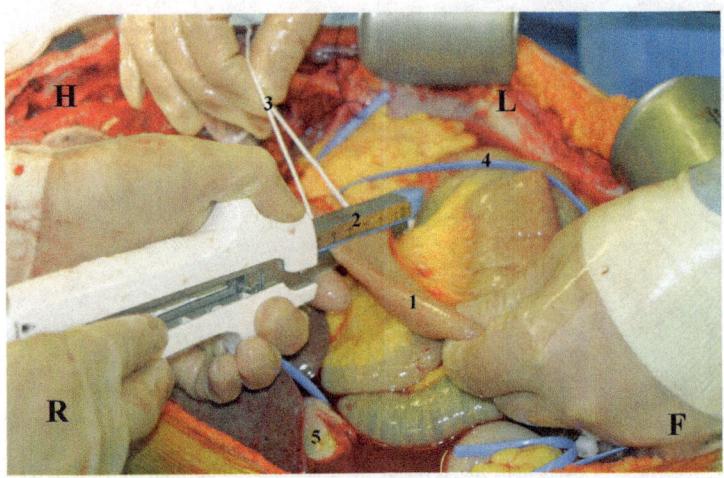

Fig. 15.3 Dividing duodenum from jejunum. 1 – Jejunum, 2 – GIA, 3 – Vessel loop between duodenum and the jejunum (white), 4 – Blue vessel loop at the pylorus level, 5 – Gallbladder emptied and flushed, *H – head, F – feet, R – right, L – left*

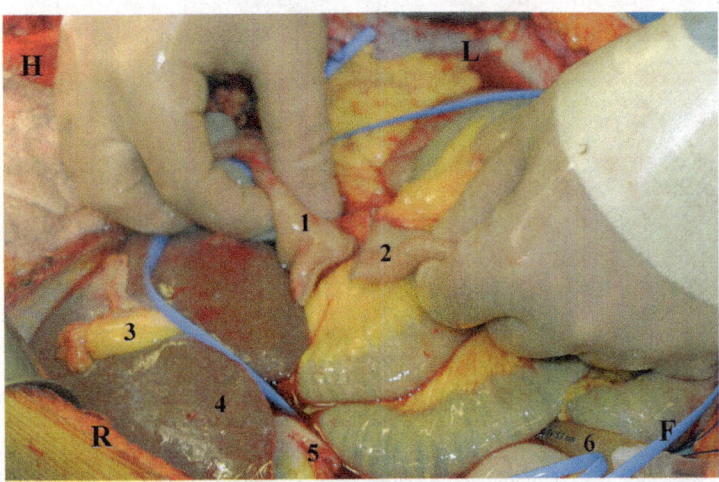

Fig. 15.4 Duodenum divided from the jejunum. 1 – Duodenum, 2 – Jejunum, 3 – Treitz ligament, 4 – Liver, *H – head, F – feet, R – right, L – left*

15.2 Pancreas, Liver and Kidneys Procurement Surgical Technique

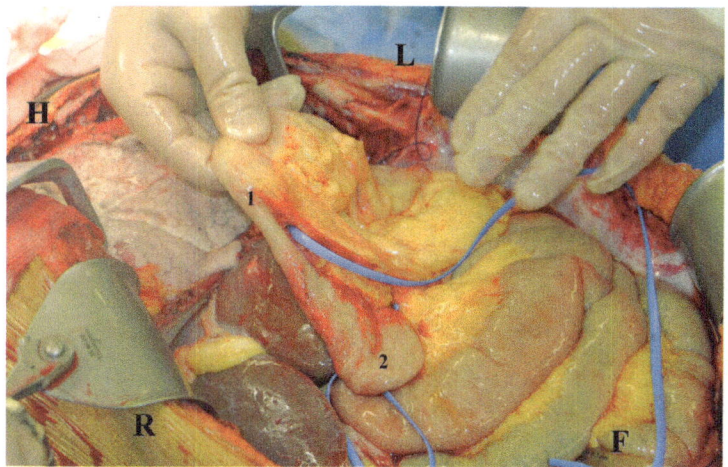

Fig. 15.5 1 – Stomach tube replaced to the duodenum, 2 – Duodenum, *H – head, F – feet, R – right, L – left*

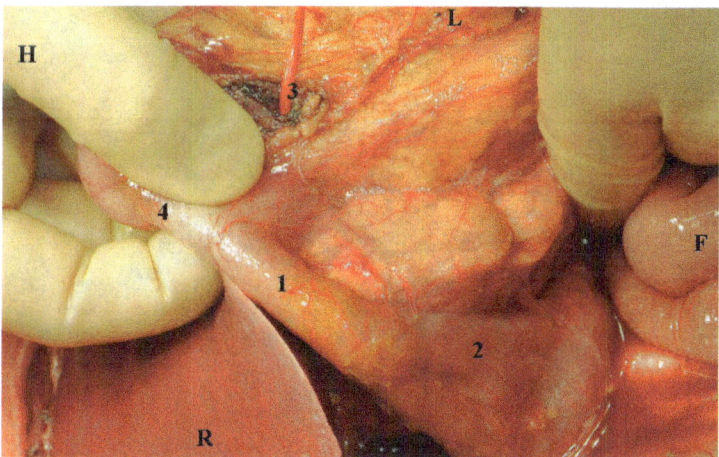

Fig. 15.6 1 – Gastric tube, 2 – Duodenum, 3 – Vessel loop at the pylorus level between pancreas and the pylorus, 4 – Pylorus, *H – head, F – feet, R – right, L – left*

3. Ask the anaesthesiologist or the transplant coordinator to inject through the gastric tube 20–80 mL povidone iodine in water solution (Fig. 15.7), together with amphotericin B (Fig. 15.8).

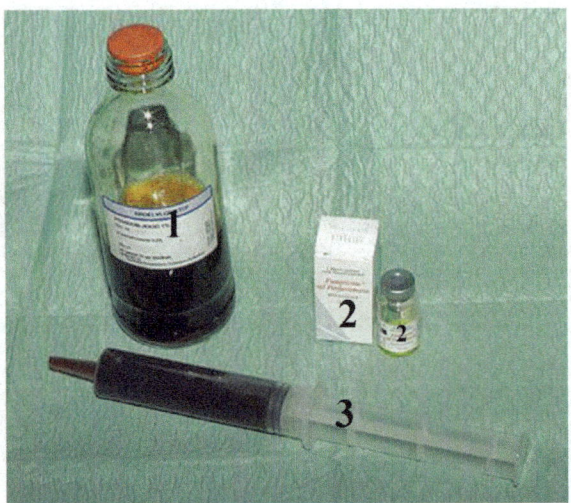

Fig. 15.7 1 – Povidone iodine in water solution, 2 – Amphotericin B, 3 – Syringe with povidone iodine in water solution

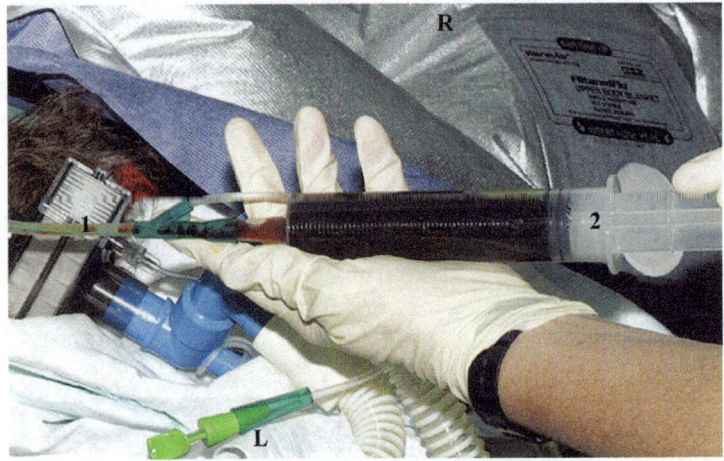

Fig. 15.8 1 – Gastric tube, 2 – Syringe with povidone iodine in water solution, *R – right*, *L – left*

15.2.3 Dividing Duodenum from the Stomach

1. Replace the gastric tube from the duodenum to the stomach.
2. Close and cut the duodenum at the level of the pylorus – use GIA for it (Figs. 15.9 and 15.10).

15.2 Pancreas, Liver and Kidneys Procurement Surgical Technique

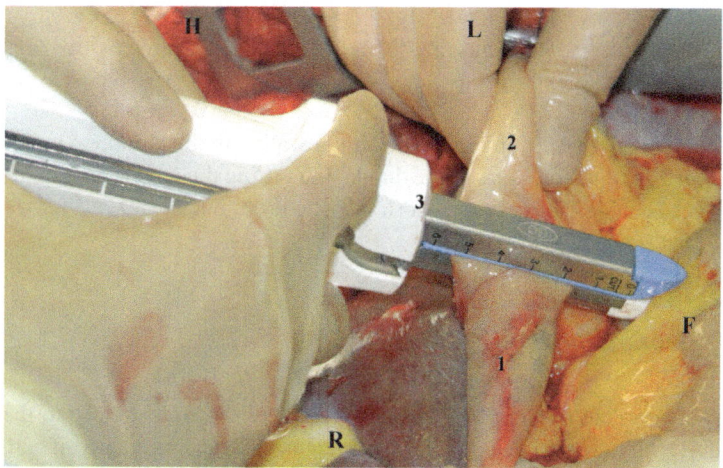

Fig. 15.9 1 – Duodenum, 2 – Stomach, 3 – GIA, *H – head, F – feet, R – right, L – left*

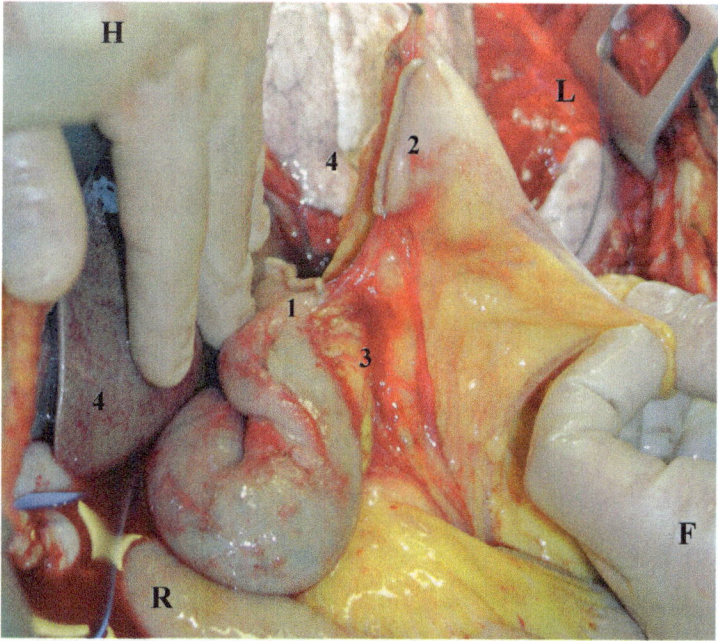

Fig. 15.10 Closed duodenum at the level of the pyrolus. 1 – Filled duodenum with povidone iodine in water solution, 2 – Pylorus, 3 – Liver, *H – head, F – feet, R – right, L – left*

ATTENTION!
- After closing, check distention of the duodenum – closing with two fingers should be possible without any tension to stick the anterior and posterior duodenum walls together.
- Avoid too much distention of the duodenum wall with the povidone iodine water solution. Too much pressure in the duodenum during the cold ischemia time may cause irreversible damage of mucosa and stapler line leakage.

15.2.4 Stomach Mobilisation

1. With scissors, cut the hepatogastric and gastrocolic ligament close to the stomach wall from the pylorus up to the oesophagus and the diaphragm on both sides: greater (Figs. 15.11 and 15.12) and lesser curvature (Figs. 15.13 and 15.14).
2. Place the mobilised stomach in the thorax (Figs. 15.15 and 15.16).

ATTENTION!
If present, save both the left aberrant hepatic artery and the left gastric artery; cut only the small branches of the left gastric artery from the side of the less curvature and also the small branches of the gastroepiploic artery coming directly into the stomach wall; stay close to the stomach wall with your scissors (Fig. 15.17).

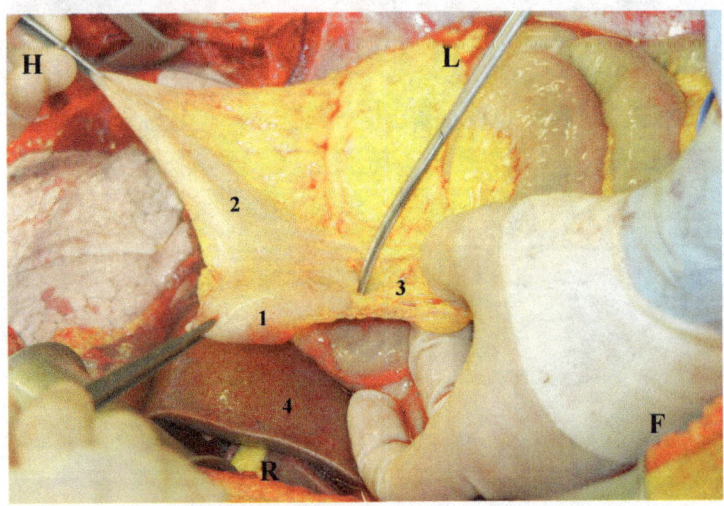

Fig. 15.11 Scissors indicate the great curvature of the stomach. 1 – Pylorus, 2 – Stomach, 3 – Gastrocolic ligament, 4 – Liver, *H – head, F – feet, R – right, L – left*

15.2 Pancreas, Liver and Kidneys Procurement Surgical Technique

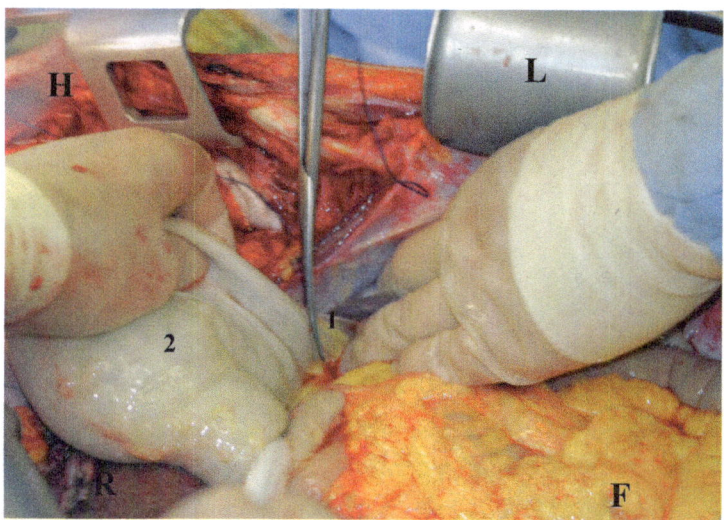

Fig. 15.12 1– The rest of the gastrocolic ligament, 2 – Stomach, *H – head, F – feet, R – right, L – left*

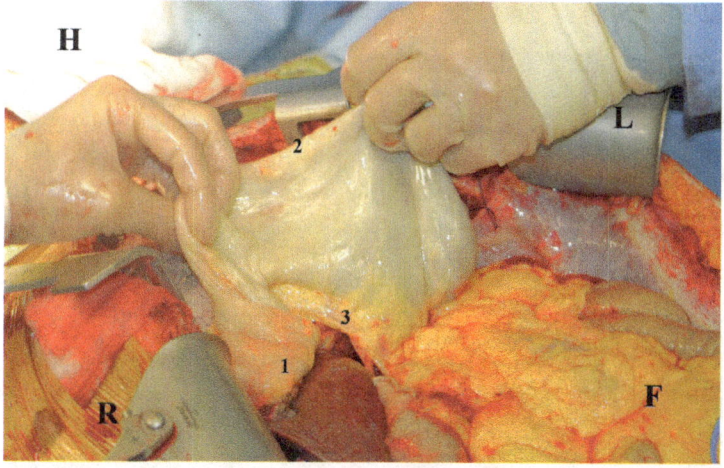

Fig. 15.13 Greater curvature is totally freed from the gastrocolic ligament. 1 – Pylorus, 2 – Greater curvature, 3 – Lesser omentum, *H – head, F – feet, R – right, L – left*

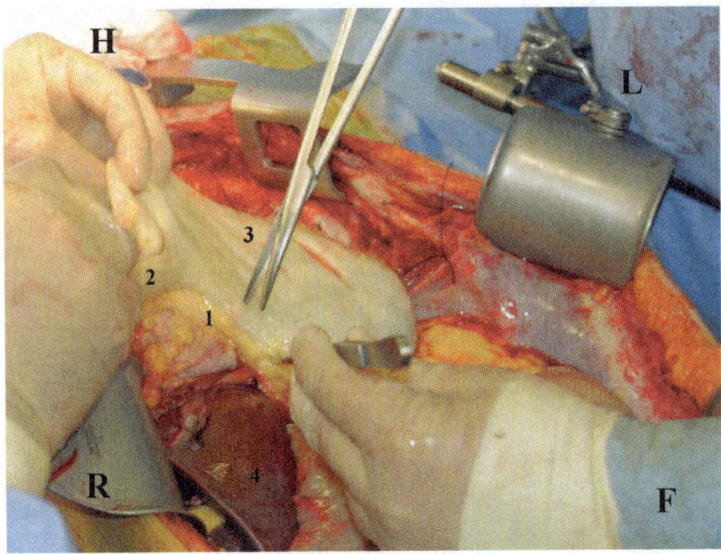

Fig. 15.14 1 – Lesser curvature of the stomach and lesser omentum, 2 – Pylorus, 3 – Stomach posterior wall, 4 – Liver, *H – head, F – feet, R – right, L – left*

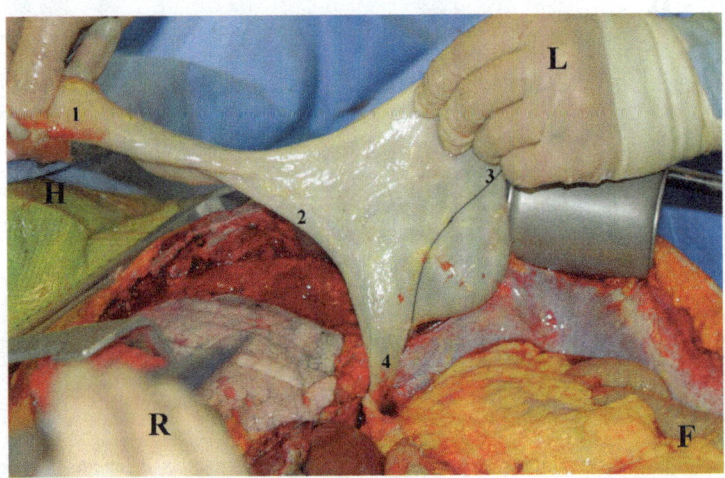

Fig. 15.15 Completely dissected stomach. 1 – Pylorus, 2 – Lesser curvature of the stomach, 3 – Greater curvature of the stomach, 4 – Oesophagus, *H – head, F – feet, R – right, L – left*

15.2 Pancreas, Liver and Kidneys Procurement Surgical Technique

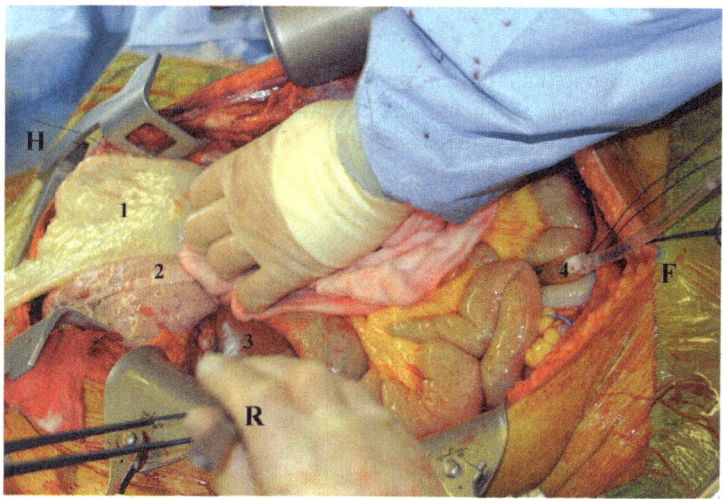

Fig. 15.16 1 – Totally mobilised stomach placed in the thorax. 2 – Right lung, 3 – Liver, 4 – Aortic cannula, *H – head, F – feet, R – right, L – left*

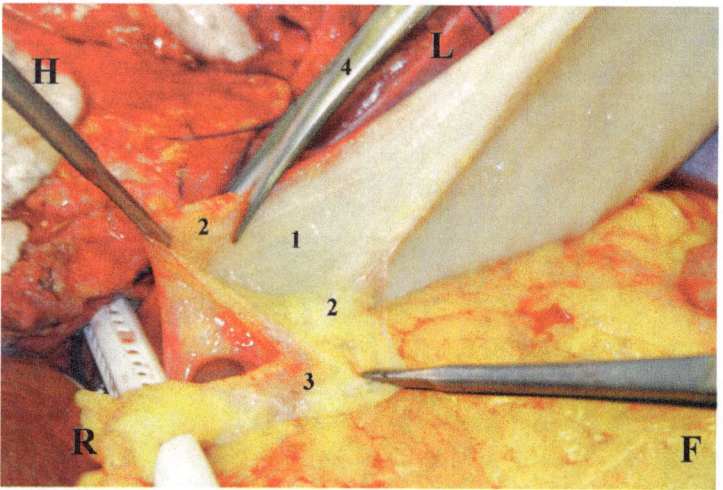

Fig. 15.17 To save the left aberrant hepatic artery, the lesser omentum is cut with the scissors close to the stomach wall. 1 – Stomach wall less curvature, 2 – Small branches of the left gastric artery to the stomach wall, 3 – Less omentum, 4 – Scissor, *H – head, F – feet, R – right, L – left*

15.2.5 Placing Small Bowel and the Colon Outside the Abdomen

1. Gently pull down in the inferior direction (towards the feet) the transverse colon together with the greater omentum to achieve optimal visualisation of the transverse mesocolon and the pancreas (Figs. 15.18 and 15.19).

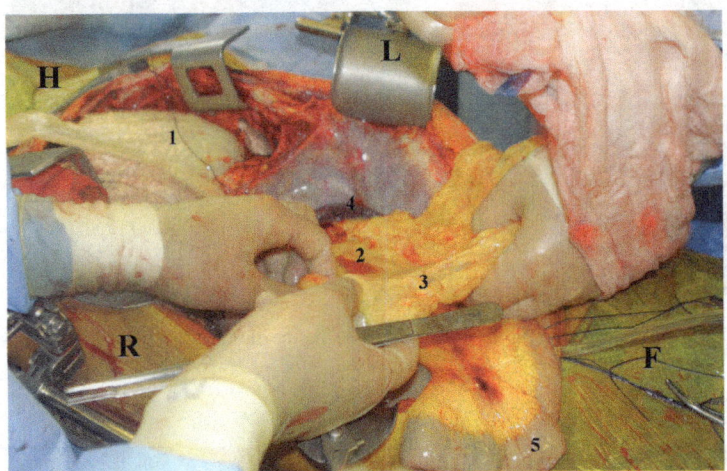

Fig. 15.18 Pulling down the greater omentum. 1 – Mobilised stomach, 2 – Pancreas, 3 – Transverse colon, 4 – Spleen, 5 – Small bowel, *H – head, F – feet, R – right, L – left* (view from the right side)

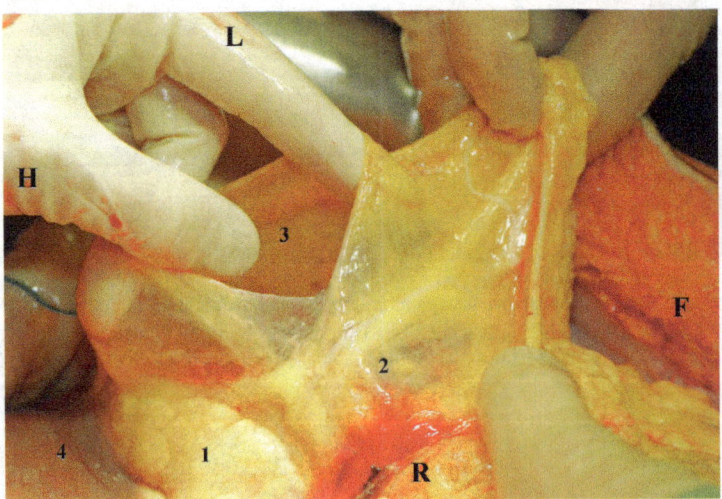

Fig. 15.19 1 – Pancreas, 2 – Transverse mesocolon, 3 – Transparent place in the transverse mesocolon, 4 – Greater omentum, *H – head, F – feet, R – right, L – left* (view from the left side)

15.2 Pancreas, Liver and Kidneys Procurement Surgical Technique

2. Look at the left side of transverse mesocolon, and try to find its transparent or thinnest avascular place and make a small hole in it with scissors.
3. Through the opening, localise the closed duodenum at the level of the Treitz ligament (Fig. 15.20).
4. In the direction to the right side, until the root of the small bowel mesentery from the opening cut the right side of the transverse mesocolon 2–3 cm beneath the lower part of the pancreas (GIA stapling device – 55 mm) (Figs. 15.21 and 15.22).

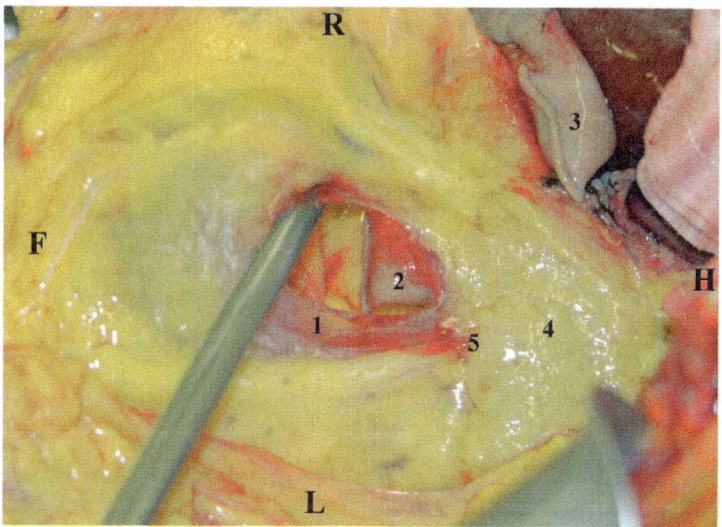

Fig. 15.20 1 – Transparent place in the transverse mesocolon, 2 – Closed duodenum at the level of the Treitz ligament, 3 – Closed duodenum at the level of the pylorus, 4 – Pancreas, 5 – Border between pancreas and transverse colon, *H – head, F – feet, R – right, L – left*

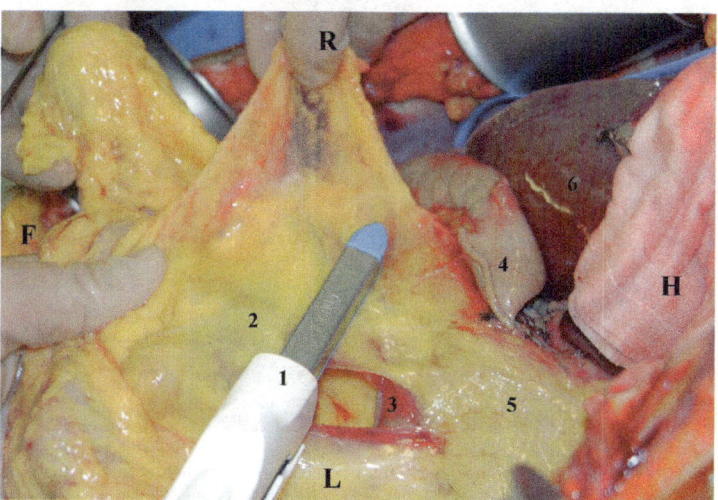

Fig. 15.21 1 – GIA, 2 – transverse mesocolon, 3 – Duodenum, 4 – Pancreas, 5 – Transverse colon, 6 – Liver, *H – head, F – feet, R – right, L – left*

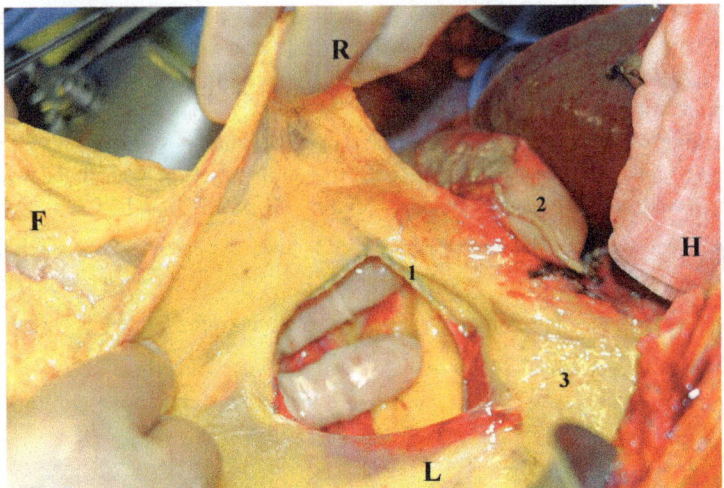

Fig. 15.22 1 – Divided transverse mesocolon, 2 – Duodenum, 3 – Pancreas, *H – head, F – feet, R – right, L – left*

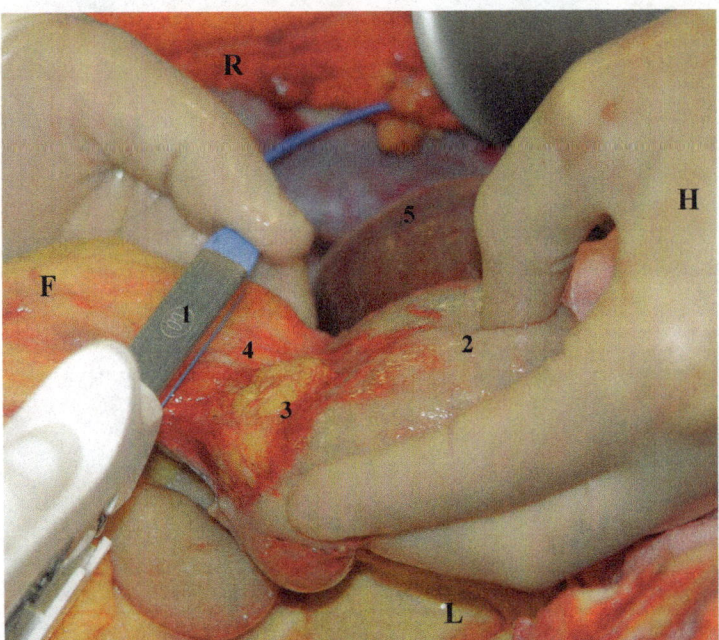

Fig. 15.23 Closing and cutting the root of small bowel mesentery below the uncinate process of the pancreas. 1 – GIA, 2 – Duodenum, 3 – Pancreas uncinate process, 4 – Root of the small bowel mesentery, *H – head, F – feet, R – right, L – left*

15.2 Pancreas, Liver and Kidneys Procurement Surgical Technique

5. Divide the root of the small bowel mesentery 3–5 cm below the uncinate process of the pancreas by using the gastrointestinal or vascular stapling device. Use several steps with a 55-mm-long stapler to do this (Figs. 15.23 and 15.24).
6. With GIA or with scissors, cut the left side of the transverse mesocolon (Figs. 15.25 and 15.26), and with the scissors, the splenocolic and phrenicocolic

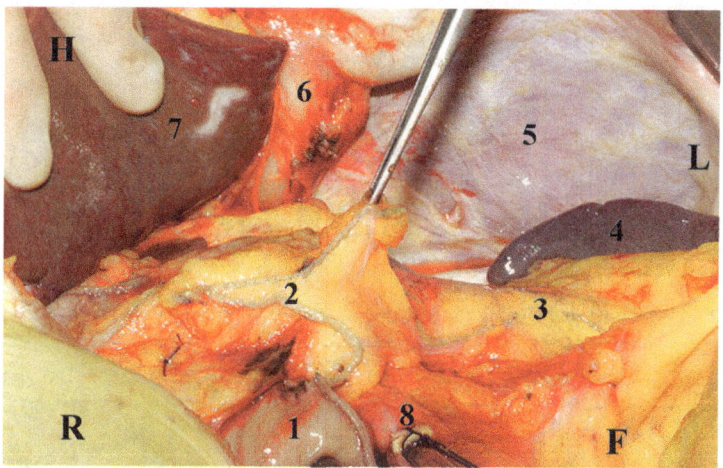

Fig. 15.24 1 – Duodenum horizontal part, 2 – Multiple closures of the root of the small bowel mesentery, 3 – Pancreas, 4 – Spleen, 5 – Diaphragm, 6 – Oesophagus, 7 – Liver, 8 – Aorta cannula, *H – head, F – feet, R – right, L – left*

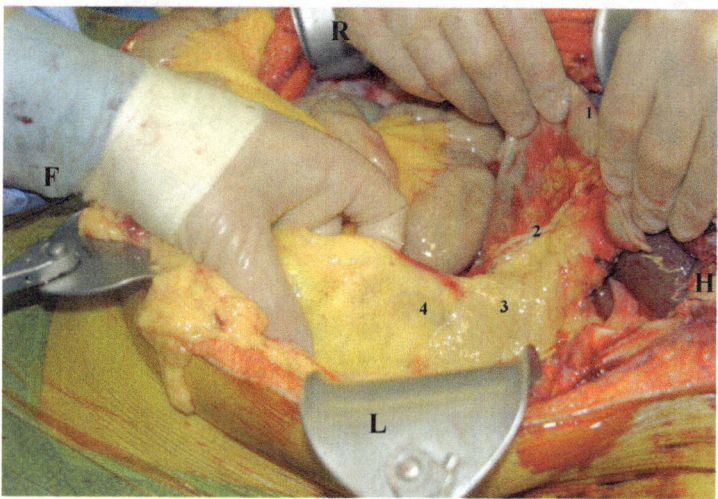

Fig. 15.25 1 – Duodenum, 2 – Closed root of the small bowel mesentery, 3 – Pancreas, 4 – Left side of the transverse mesocolon, *H – head, F – feet, R – right, L – left*

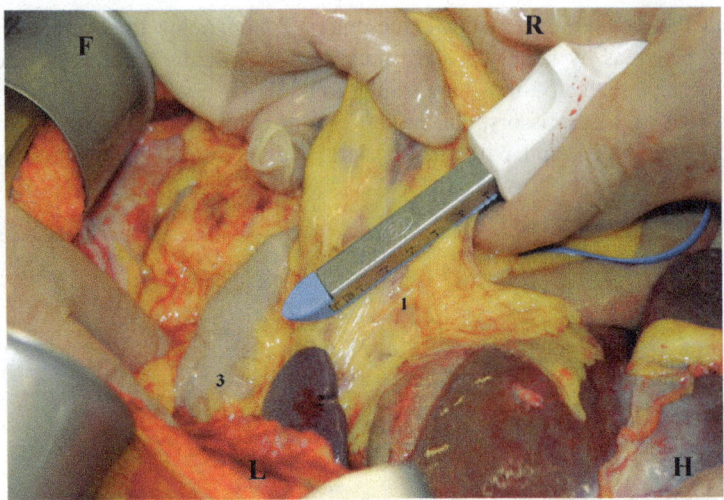

Fig. 15.26 1 – Cutting and closing the left side of transverse mesocolon with GIA, 2 – Spleen, 3 – Spleen flexure of the colon, H – head, F – feet, R – right, L – left

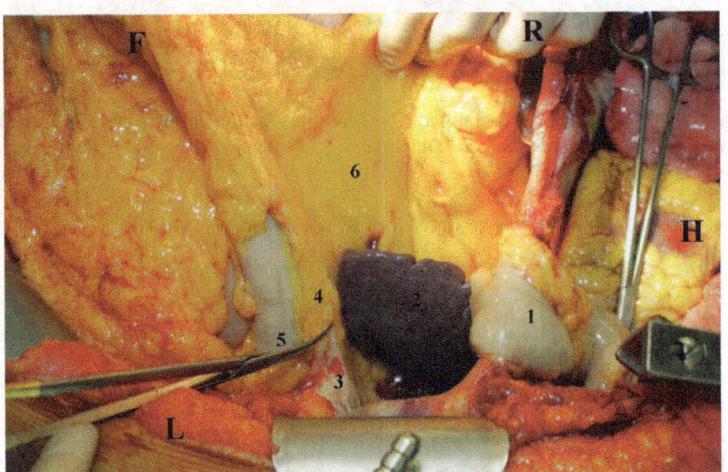

Fig. 15.27 Mobilisation of the splenic flexure of the colon. 1 – Stomach, 2 – Spleen, 3 – Splenocolic ligament, 4 –Splenic flexure of the colon already cut, 5 – Descending colon, 6 – Transverse mesocolon, H – head, F – feet, R – right, L – left

ligament until the descending colon (Figs. 15.27 and 15.28). The left side of the colon transverse mesentery, below the pancreas, is almost avascular.

7. Free the descending colon up to the sigmoid (Fig. 15.29); move the entire specimen, which now consists of the small bowel and the colon outside abdomen, and place it on the donor legs (Figs. 15.30 and 15.31). Now, the pancreas, liver and the two kidneys remain in the abdomen.

15.2 Pancreas, Liver and Kidneys Procurement Surgical Technique

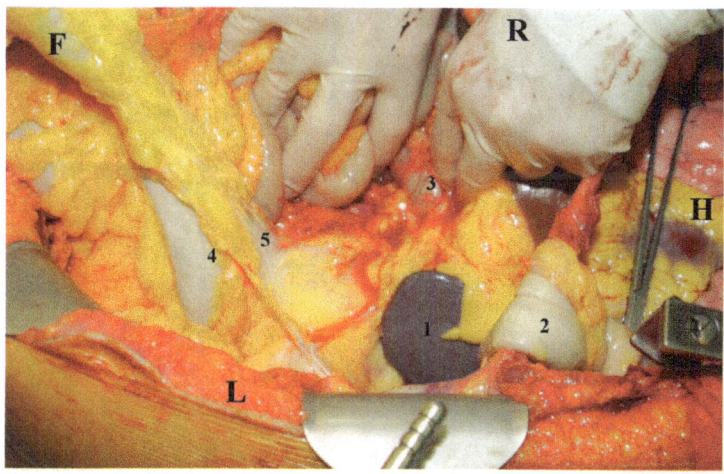

Fig. 15.28 1 – Spleen, 2 – Stomach, 3 – Duodenum (horizontal part), 4 – Descending colon, 5 – Mesocolon, *H – head, F – feet, R – right, L – left*

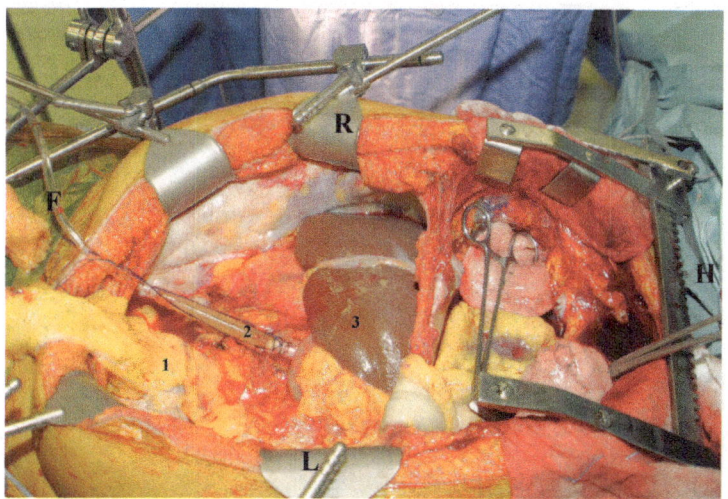

Fig. 15.29 1 – Sigmoid, 2 – Aortic cannula, 3 – Liver, *H – head, F – feet, R – right, L – left*

ATTENTION!

- Take small steps and take small amounts of tissues between the stapling device jaws (Fig. 15.24).

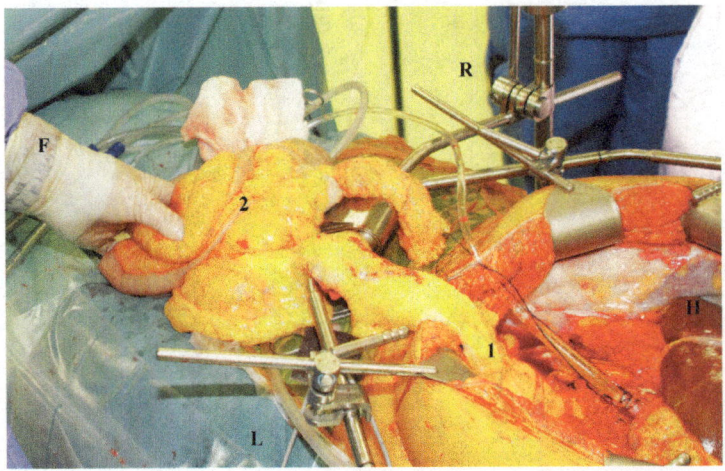

Fig. 15.30 1 – Sigmoid, 2 – Small bowel and colon outside the abdomen, *H – head, F – feet, R – right, L – left*

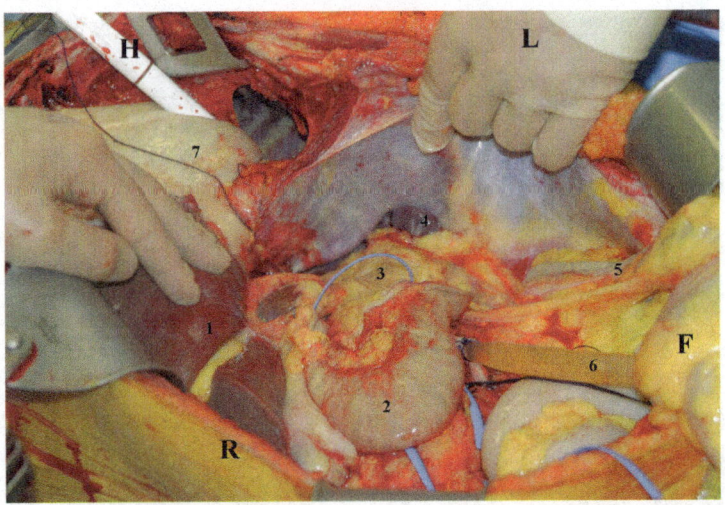

Fig. 15.31 1 – Liver, 2 – Duodenum, 3 – Pancreas, 4 – Spleen, 5 – Sigmoid, 6 – Aorta cannula, 7 – Stomach, *H – head, F – feet, R – right, L – left*

- Close the jaws of the stapling device very slowly to adapt the tissue and the stapling device for efficient closing and cutting.
- Always use appropriate staplers for the appropriate tissues.

15.3 Pancreas and Liver Vascular Splitting (8–13)

15.3.1 Surgical Steps

1. Cut the gastroduodenal artery 0.3–0.4 mm beneath the common hepatic artery (Fig. 15.32), after cutting half the diameter of the gastroduodenal artery. Mark it now, or cut it totally and mark it before packing the pancreatic side of this artery with Prolene (Ethicon) 5/0 suture. Remember that after procurement it can be very difficult to find the splenic artery deep in the pancreas parenchyma.
2. Dissect the common hepatic artery, first 0.5 cm of the splenic artery and celiac trunk towards aorta, (Figs. 15.33 and 15.34). Look for the dorsal pancreatic artery, arising from the common hepatic artery or the celiac trunk; do not cut it. Save it.
3. Cut the portal vein 2–3 cm above the pancreas head (Figs. 15.35 and 15.36) and mark it with a thin nonabsorbable surgical suture.
4. Cut the splenic artery 0.2–0.3 cm from the celiac trunk (Fig. 15.37).
5. Cut half the diameter of the splenic artery; mark it now, or cut it totally and mark it before packing the pancreatic side of the artery with Prolene (Ethicon) 5/0 suture. Remember that after procurement it can be very difficult to find it in the pancreas parenchyma.

ATTENTION!
- If you procure the pancreas for transplantation during vessel dissection, never cut any artery arising from the common hepatic artery, celiac trunk or splenic artery to the pancreas. By cutting you will damage the dorsal pancreatic artery

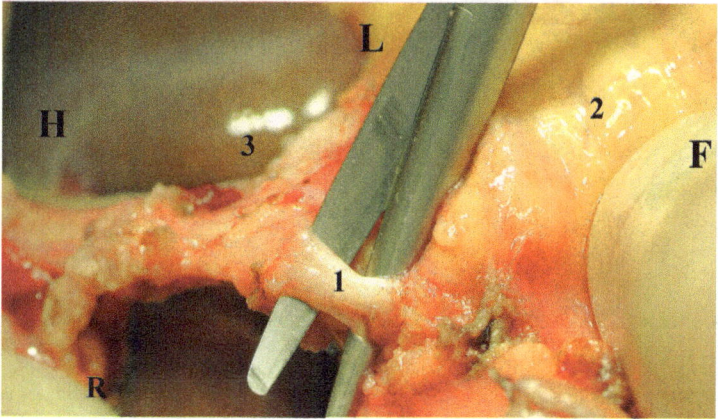

Fig. 15.32 Vascular dissection of the hepatoduodenal ligament. 1 – Gastroduodenal artery, 2 – Pancreas, 3 – Liver, *H – head, F – feet, R – right, L – left*

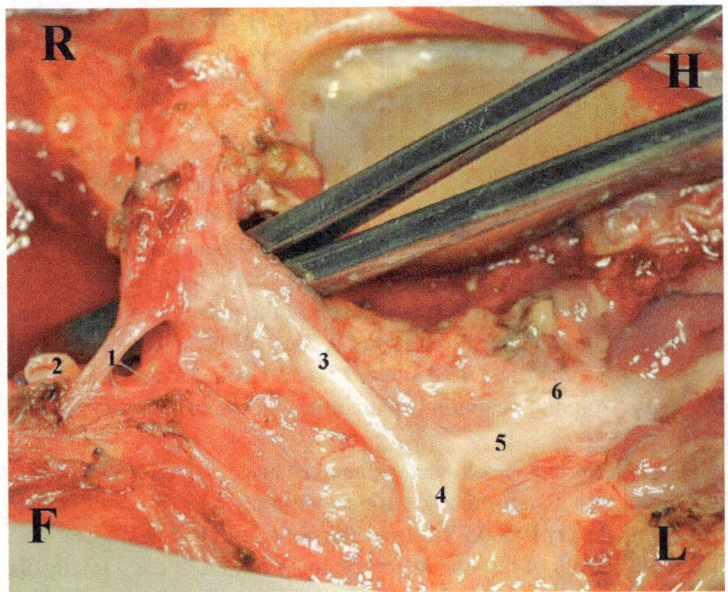

Fig. 15.33 1 – Gastroduodenal artery, 2 – Distal part of the CBD, 3 – Common hepatic artery, 4 – Splenic artery, 5 – Celiac trunk, 6 – Cut-off left gastric artery, *H – head, F – feet, R – right, L – left*

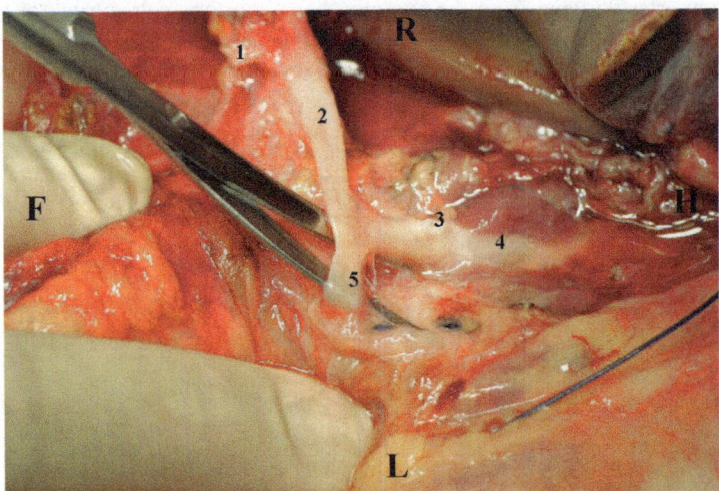

Fig. 15.34 1 – Stump of the gastroduodenal artery, 2 – Common hepatic artery, 3 – Stump of the left gastric artery, 4 – Celiac trunk, 5 – Splenic artery, *H – head, F – feet, R – right, L – left*

15.3 Pancreas and Liver Vascular Splitting

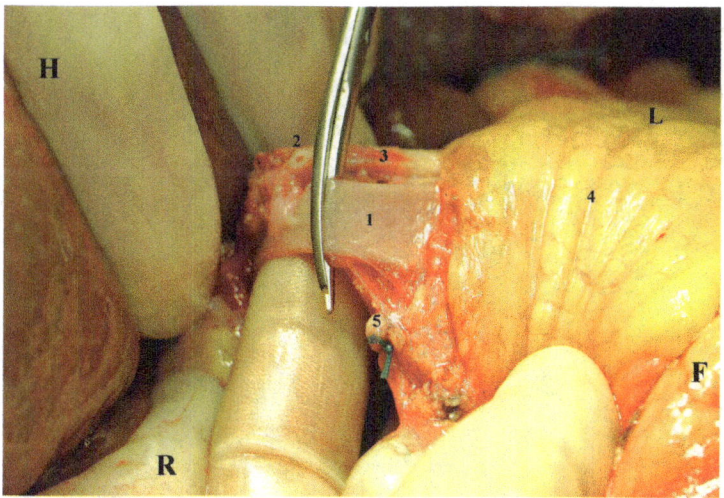

Fig. 15.35 1 – Portal vein, 2 – Cut gastroduodenal artery, 3 – Common hepatic artery, 4 – Pancreas, 5 – Ligated distal common bile duct, *H – head, F – feet, R – right, L – left*

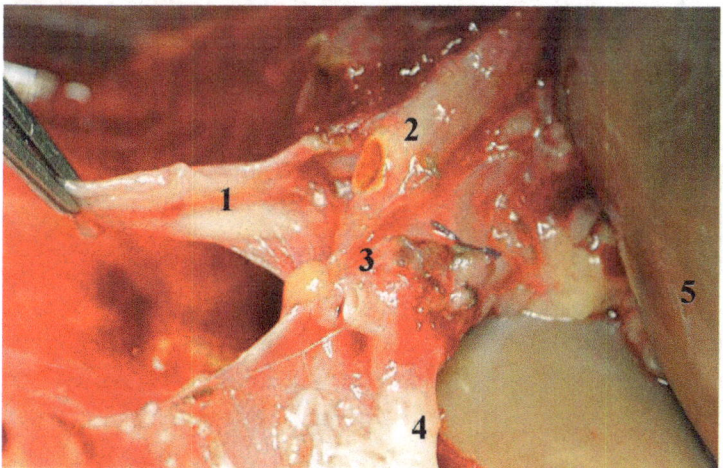

Fig. 15.36 1 – Portal vein, 2 – Common bile duct, 3 – Gastroduodenal artery, 4 – Common hepatic artery, 5 – Left liver lobe

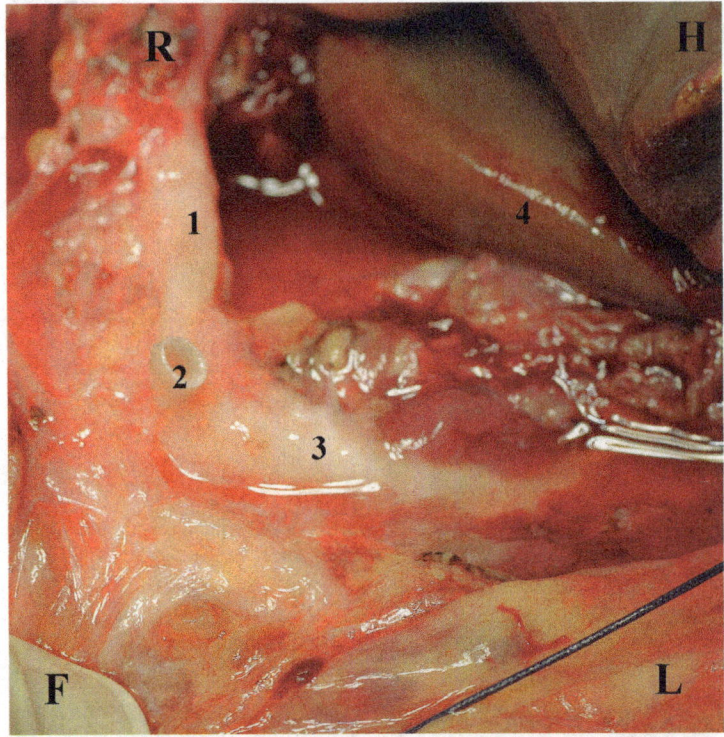

Fig. 15.37 1 – Common hepatic artery, 2 – Stump of the splenic artery, 3 – Celiac trunk, 4 – Caudate liver lobe

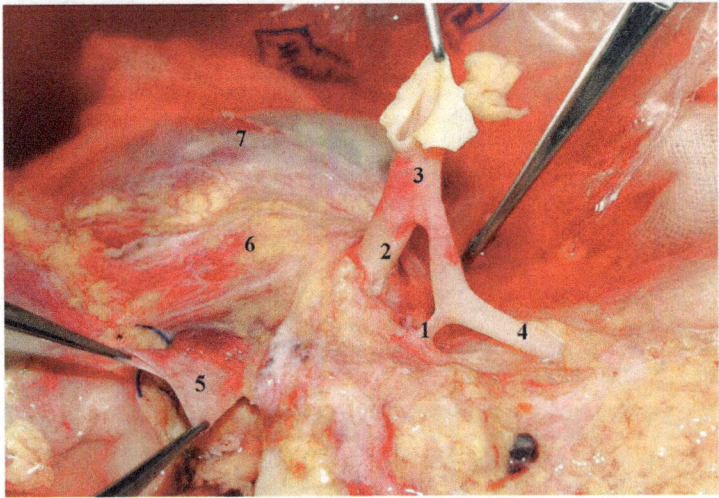

Fig. 15.38 1 – Dorsal pancreatic artery, 2 – Common hepatic artery, 3 – Celiac trunk, 4 – Splenic artery, 5 – Portal vein, 6 – Pancreas head, 7 – Duodenum

15.3 Pancreas and Liver Vascular Splitting

and in this case the pancreas might not be useful for transplantation (Fig. 15.38).

- In presence of the right aberrant hepatic artery, with a complete extra-pancreatic course, one can decide to dissect the artery from the posterior side of the pancreas head close to its origin with a 1-cm cuff or patch from the SMA or if it is impossible (high-risk pancreas capsule injury) cut the right aberrant hepatic artery close to the pancreatic head. Before cutting, consider the best possibility of arterial reconstruction (read the next point).
- In case of an intra-pancreatic course of the right aberrant hepatic artery (very rare) (Fig. 15.39), its division should be done after consultation between pancreas and liver transplant teams. If this artery is cut close to the pancreatic head, the liver surgeon must have the possibility to implant the stump of the right aberrant hepatic artery into the ostium of either the gastroduodenal or the splenic artery (Fig. 15.40).
- In case of a dorsal pancreatic artery arising from the common hepatic artery or from the celiac trunk the procurement surgeon is obliged to consult with the liver and the pancreas acceptor centre(s).

In this case, the celiac trunk and the SMA on the one aortic patch have to be given to the pancreas, and the common hepatic artery has to be cut 3–5 mm from the celiac trunk (Fig. 15.41).

- Possibilities of vascular pancreas and liver splitting (black bars) in order to make both organs transplantable (Fig. 15.42)

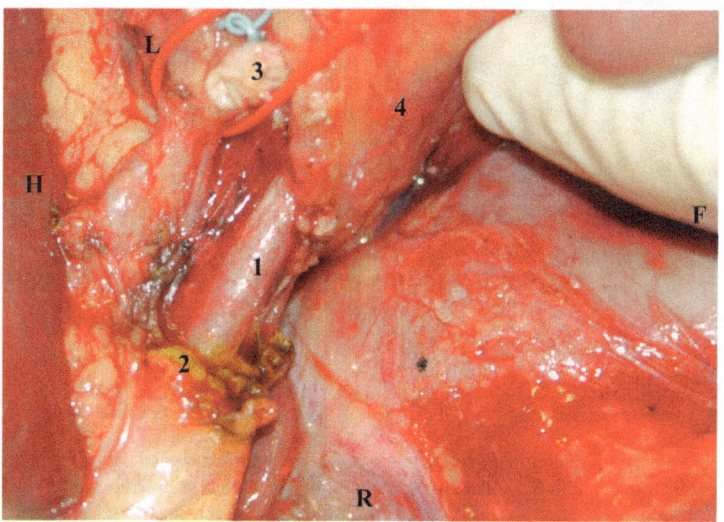

Fig. 15.39 Right aberrant hepatic artery, 2 – Cut proximal part of the ductus choledochus, 3 – Ligated distal part of common bile duct, 4 – Pancreas head posterior side, *H – head, F – feet, R – right, L – left*

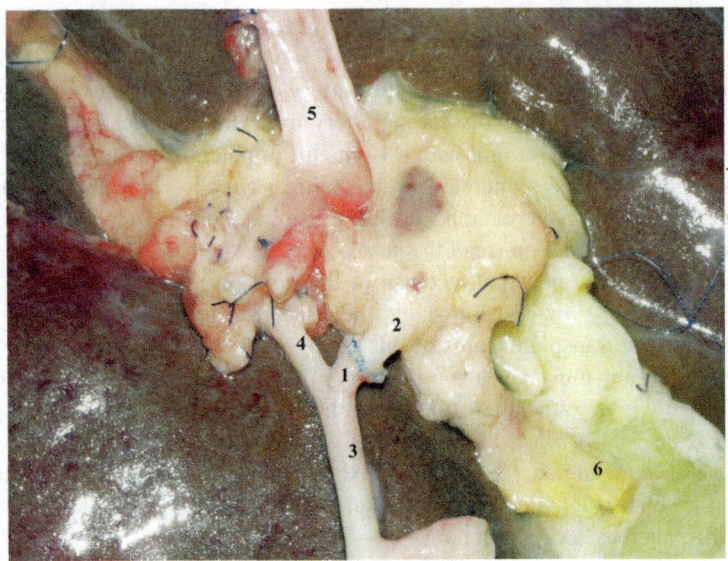

Fig. 15.40 Hilum of the liver. 1 – Gastroduodenal artery, 2 – Right aberrant hepatic artery (*"end to end"* anastomose), 3 – Common hepatic artery, 4 – Proper hepatic artery, 5 – Portal vein, 6 – CBD

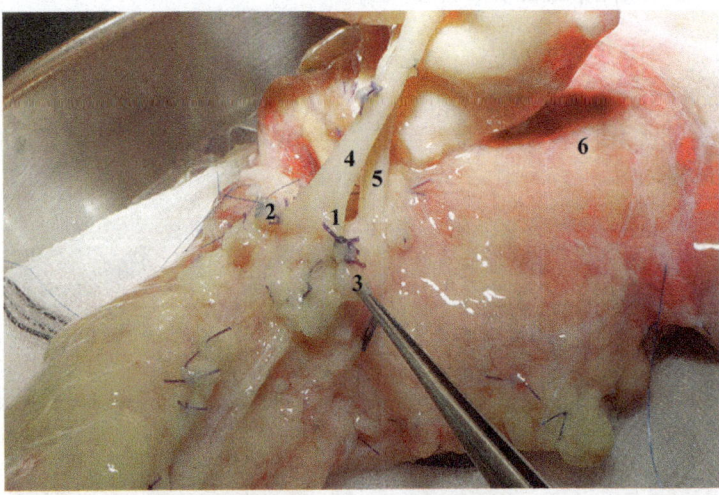

Fig. 15.41 Pancreas procured with celiac trunk and SMA with aorta patch. 1 – Dorsal pancreatic artery arising from the celiac trunk, 2 – Sutured stump of common hepatic artery, 3 – Ligated stump of the splenic artery, 4 – Celiac trunk, 5 – SMA, 6 – Pancreas head - posterior side

15.3 Pancreas and Liver Vascular Splitting

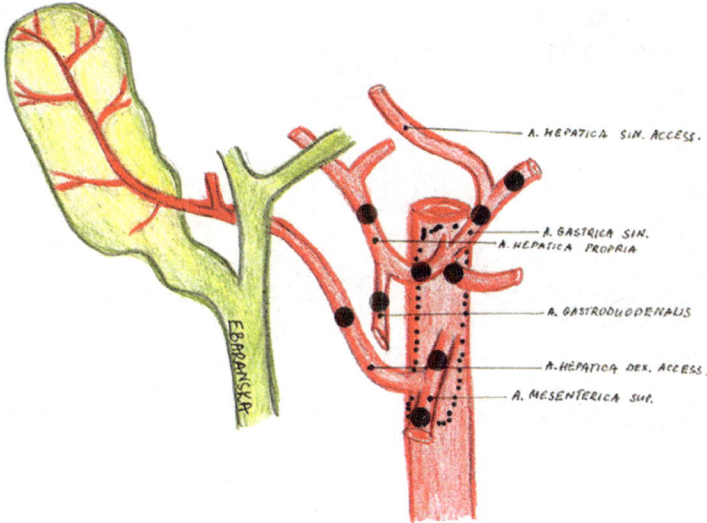

Fig. 15.42 Possibilities of the vascular arterial splitting between the pancreas and the liver to make both organs suitable for transplantation (black bars and dots)

- Advantages of splitting liver and pancreas in the recipient centre are as follows:
  - Decrease cold ischemia time.
  - Splitting in situ in the donor body – better anatomical orientation.
- Pancreas procurement for whole organ transplantation should be avoided in the following situations: with a very small child as a donor, especially when the liver will be given to a "difficult recipient" such as another very small child or in the case of liver retransplantation following an earlier vascular thrombosis and/or when there is a lack of – or an unsuitable – toolkit for pancreas reconstruction.

15.3.2 Pancreas Procurement

15.3.2.1 Spleen and Pancreas Tail Mobilisation: Surgical Steps

1. Mobilise the spleen by cutting through the following spleen ligaments: phrenicosplenic (Fig. 15.43) and splenorenal (Figs. 15.44 and 15.45).
2. Free the spleen and the pancreas tail from retroperitoneal attachments up to the SMA, celiac trunk and the left side of the abdominal aorta. Use the spleen as a *handle* (Figs. 15.46–15.49).

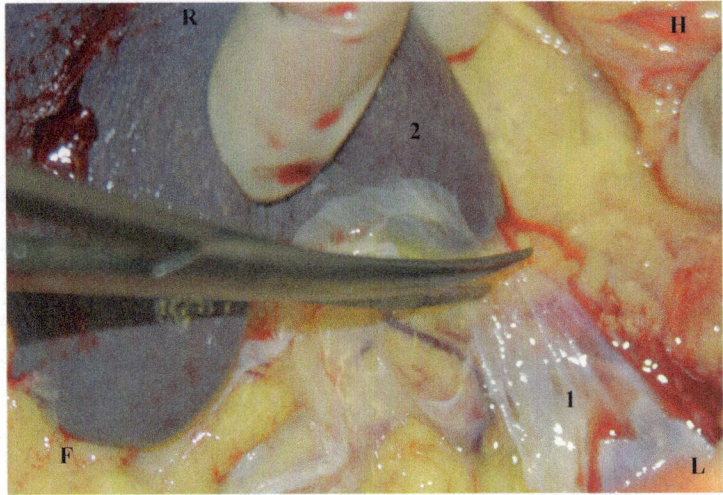

Fig. 15.43 1 – Phrenicosplenic ligament, 2 – Spleen, *H – head, F – feet, R – right, L – left*

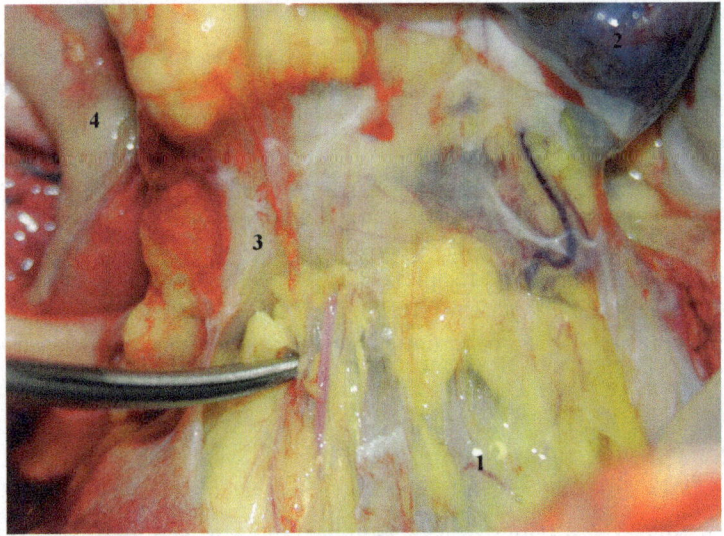

Fig. 15.44 1 – Left kidney, 2 – Spleen, 3 – Splenorenal ligament, 4 – Duodenum horizontal part

15.3 Pancreas and Liver Vascular Splitting

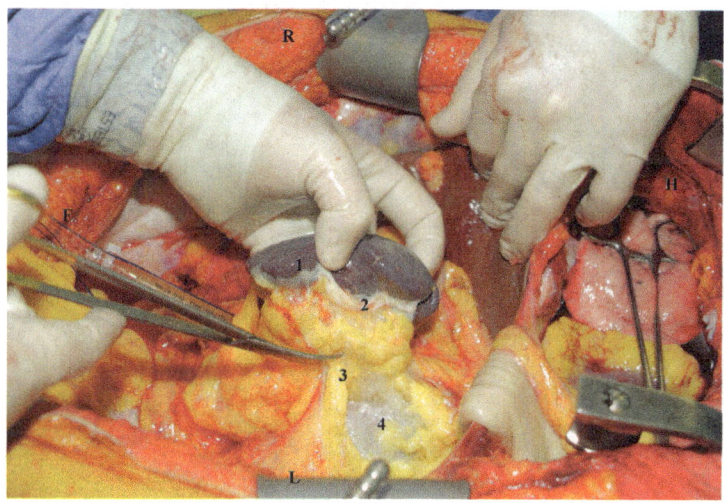

Fig. 15.45 1 – Spleen, 2 – Phrenicocolic ligament, 3 – Splenorenal ligament, 4 – Left kidney, *H – head, F – feet, R – right, L – left*

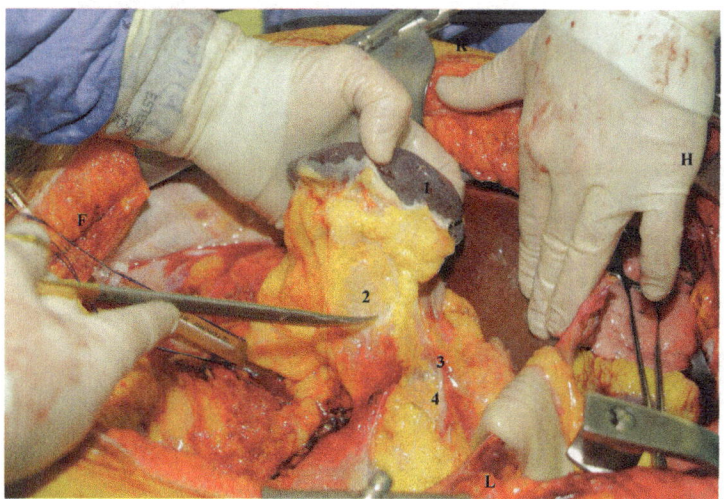

Fig. 15.46 1 – Use the spleen as a *"handle"*, 2 – Pancreas tail, 3 – Abdominal attachment of the pancreas (avascular plane anterior side of the left adrenal gland), 4 – Left adrenal gland, *H – head, F – feet, R – right, L – left*

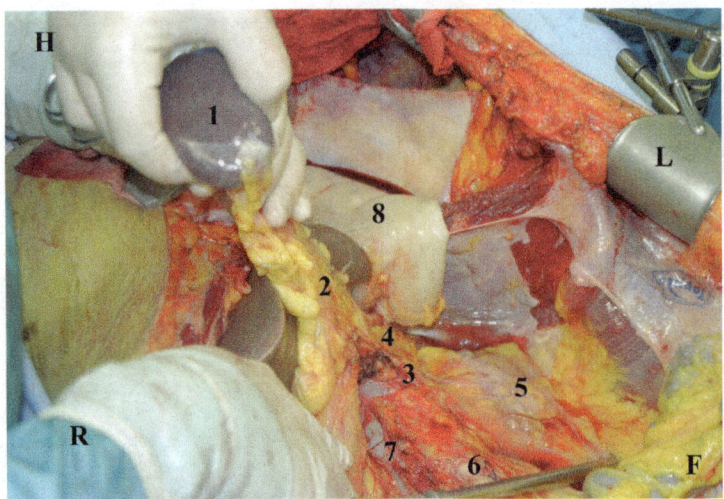

Fig. 15.47 1 – Spleen as a "handle", 2 – Pancreas tail, 3 – Left renal vein, 4 – Celiac plexus (left side), 5 – Left kidney, 6 – Abdominal aorta, 7 – Inferior vena cava (IVC), 8 – Stomach, *H – head, F – feet, R – right, L – left*

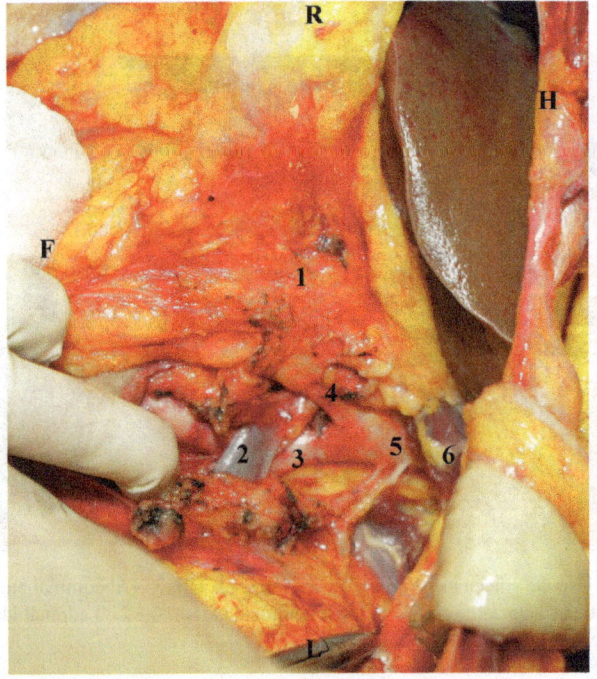

Fig. 15.48 1 – Pancreas, 2 – Left renal vein, 3 – Left renal artery, 4 – SMA, 5 – Abdominal aorta, 6 – Crural diaphragm, *H – head, F – feet, R – right, L – left*

15.3 Pancreas and Liver Vascular Splitting

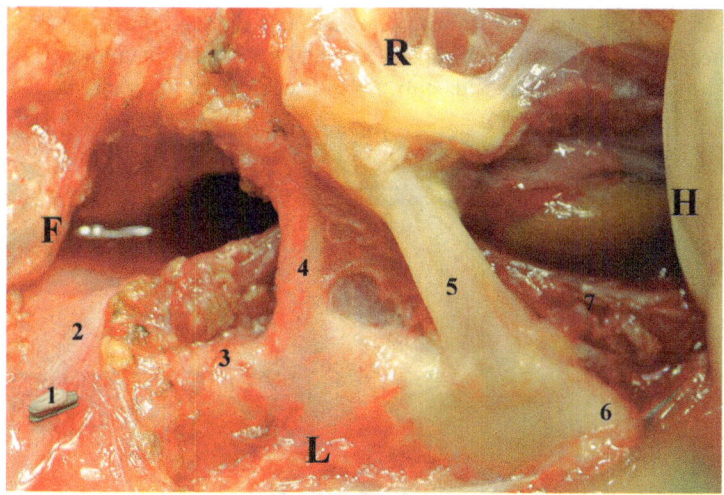

Fig. 15.49 1 – Left adrenal vein, 2 – Left renal vein, 3 – Left side of aorta, 4 – SMA, 5 – Celiac trunk, 6 – Supraceliac aorta, 7 – Right crus of diaphragma, *H – head, F – feet, R – right, L – left*

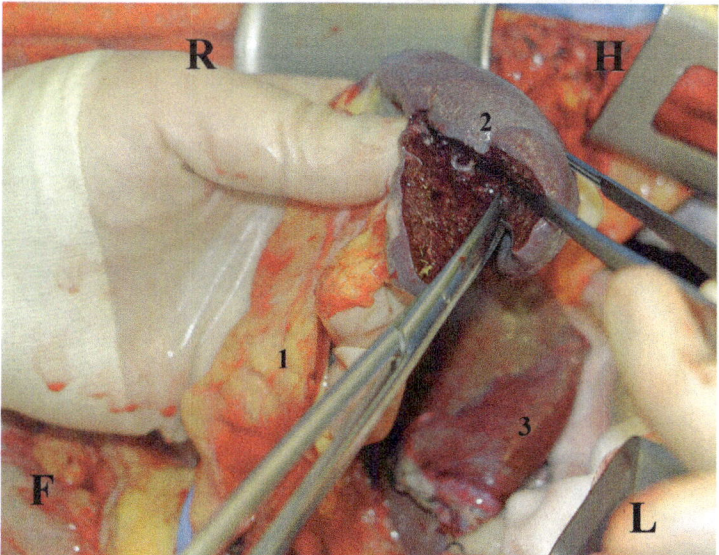

Fig. 15.50 Cutting the spleen for laboratory typing. 1 – Pancreas tail, 2 – External surface of the spleen, 3 – Liver, *H – head, F – feet, R – right, L – left*

ATTENTION!
- Because of the high risk of the pancreas tail damage, never perform total splenectomy in situ before cold perfusion and pancreas procurement.
- For the laboratory typing, cut only small piece or the external surface of the spleen (Figs. 15.50–15.52).

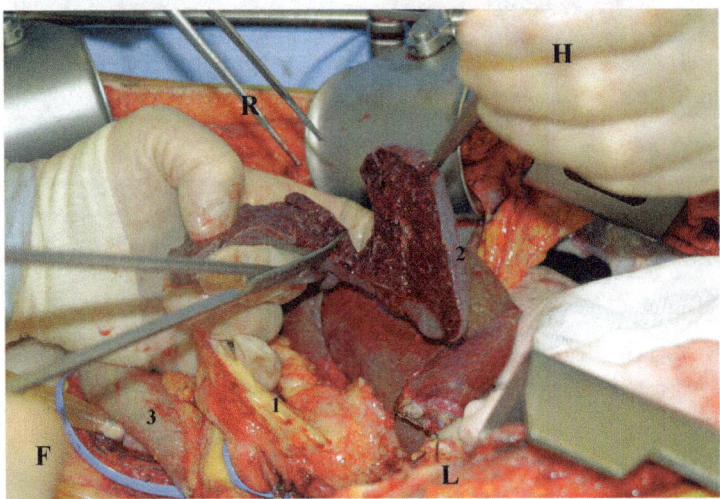

Fig. 15.51 Cutting the spleen for laboratory typing. 1 – Pancreas tail, 2 – External surface of the spleen, 3 – Duodenum, *H – head, F – feet, R – right, L – left*

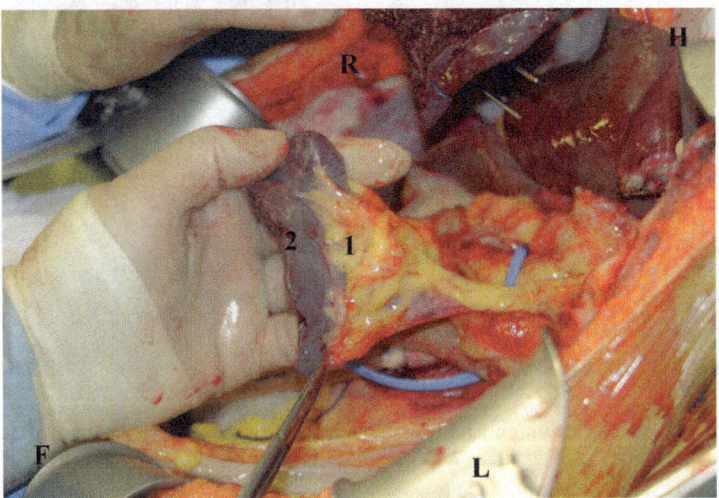

Fig. 15.52 Cutting the spleen for laboratory typing. 1 – Splenic hilum intact, 2 – Spleen without external surface, *H – head, F – feet, R – right, L – left*

15.3 Pancreas and Liver Vascular Splitting

- Always procure pancreas tail with intact hilum of the spleen (Fig. 15.53).
- Total splenectomy should be done during back-table process (Fig. 15.54) or after pancreas revascularisation in the recipient centre.

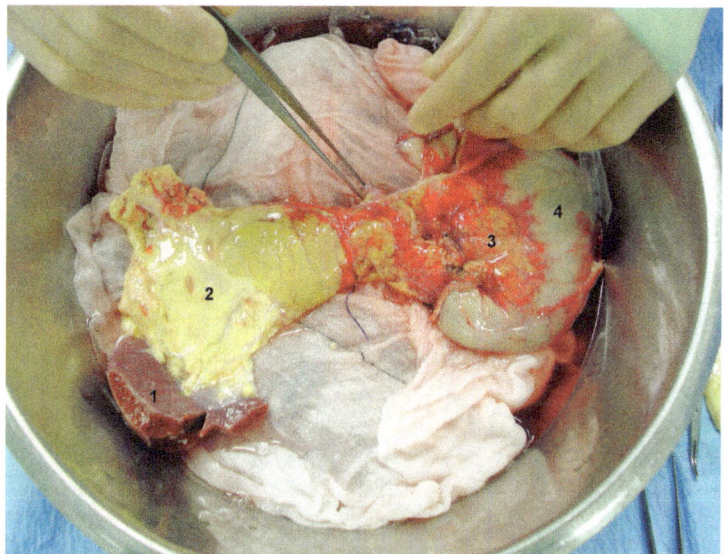

Fig. 15.53 Procured pancreas. 1 – Partial splenectomy, 2 – Splenic hilum intact, 3 – Pancreas head, 4 – Duodenum

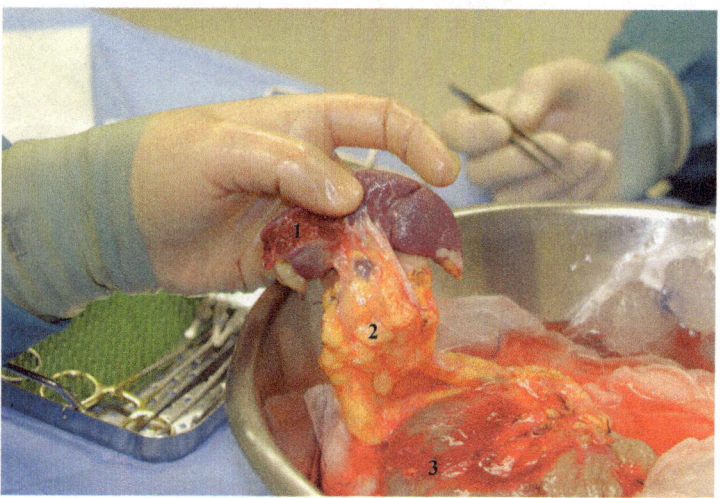

Fig. 15.54 Splenectomy during the back-table process. 1 – Spleen after partial splenectomy, 2 –Pancreas tail, 3 – Duodenum

15.3.3 Cutting SMA with Aortic Patch: In Steps

1. Dissect the superior mesenteric artery and the celiac trunk also from the right side of the aorta (finally both sides) (Fig. 15.55). At a distance of about 2.00 cm from abdominal aorta, the SMA and the celiac trunk are free of tissues.

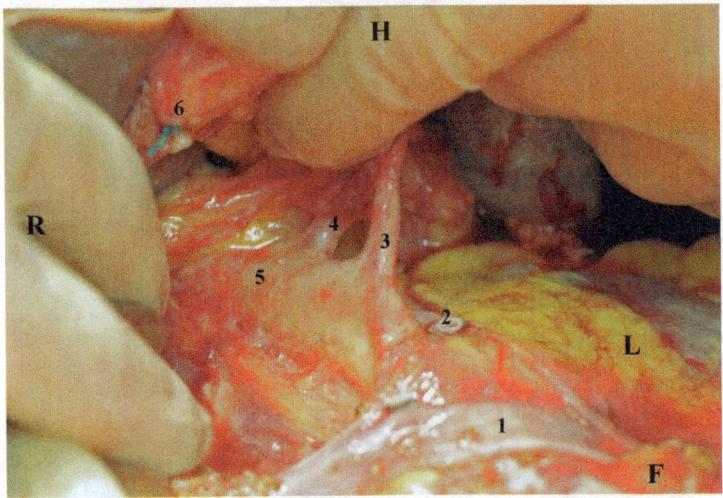

Fig. 15.55 Celiac plexus dissection around the abdominal aorta, SMA and celiac trunk. 1 – Left renal vein, 2 – Cut and closed adrenal vein, 3 – SMA, 4 – Celiac trunk, 5 – Abdominal aorta, 6 – Ligated at the superior border of the pancreas common bile duct *H – head, F – feet, R – right, L – left*

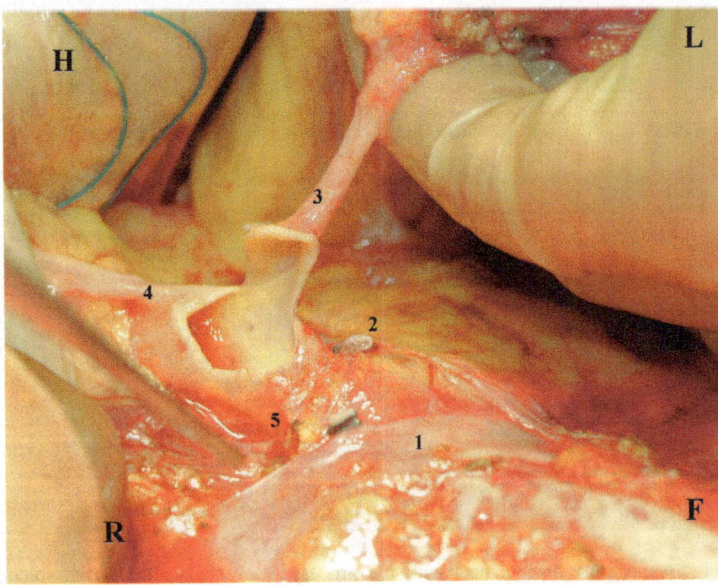

Fig. 15.56 1 – Left renal vein, 2 – Cut and closed left adrenal vein, 3 – SMA, 4 – Abdominal aorta, 5 – Region of right renal artery, *H – head, F – feet, R – right, L – left*

15.3 Pancreas and Liver Vascular Splitting

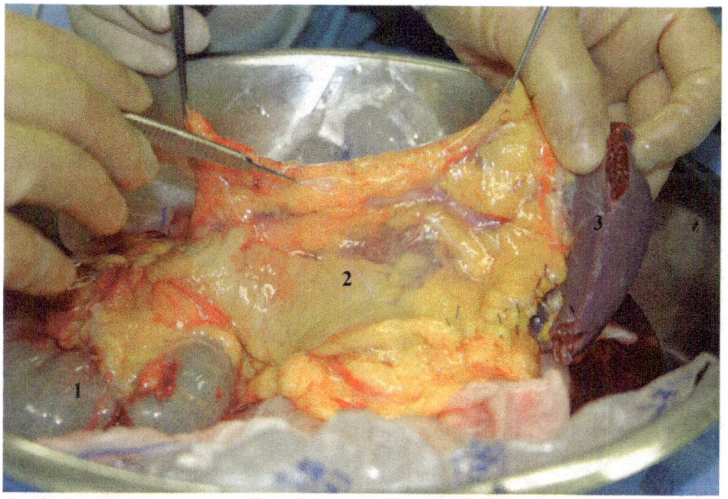

Fig. 15.57 1 – Duodenum, 2 – Pancreas, 3 – Spleen after partial splenectomy

2. Cut the SMA from the aorta with the patch. Stay away from the celiac trunk and the ostia of the renal arteries (Fig. 15.56).
3. Place the procured pancreas in a sterile container filled with ice and cold sterile 0.9% NaCl or Ringer lactate or preservation solution (Fig. 15.57).
4. Before packing, examine the pancreas one more time. Take the final decision about suitability for transplantation, mark the wall of the SMA, splenic and gastroduodenal artery with the Prolene (Ethicon) 5/0 surgical suture (Fig. 15.58).

15.3.4 Whole Pancreas Procurement for Islets Isolation: Surgical Technique

1. Pancreas should be procured following the same rules as during the procurement for whole organ transplantation: decontaminated with duodenum closed on both sides, ligated common bile duct and spleen hilum intact (Fig. 15.59) to avoid damage to the aberrant pancreatic ducts running from the head of the pancreas to the duodenum.
2. Vessels can be cut much shorter; for example, the portal vein can be cut very low at the level of superior mesenteric vein (SMV) and splenic vein (Fig. 15.60). Short cut vessels should be marked with the Prolene (Ethicon) suture 5/0. Partial splenectomy for the laboratory typing is permitted. Total splenectomy should be avoided and finally, the pancreas has to be retrieved with the spleen hilum intact and ligated common bile duct.

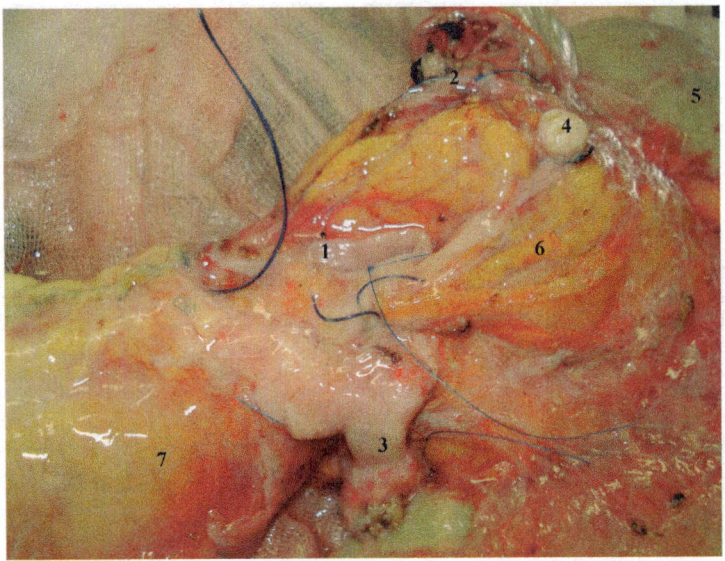

Fig. 15.58 Procured pancreas with following vessels marked with a polypropylene suture 5/0. 1 – Portal vein, 2 – Gastroduodenal artery, 3 – SMA, 4 – Ligated common bile duct, 5 – Duodenum, 6 – Pancreas head, 7 – Pancreas tail, *H – head, F – feet, R – right, L – left*

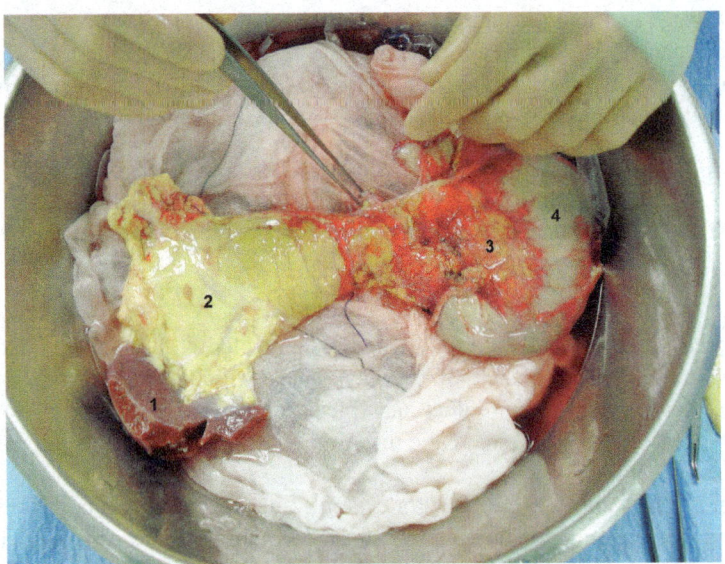

Fig. 15.59 Pancreas for islet isolation should be procured following the same rules as for transplantation. 1 – Spleen, 2 – Splenic hilum must be intact, 3 – Without damage of pancreas parenchyma, 4 – Duodenum

15.4 Liver Procurement

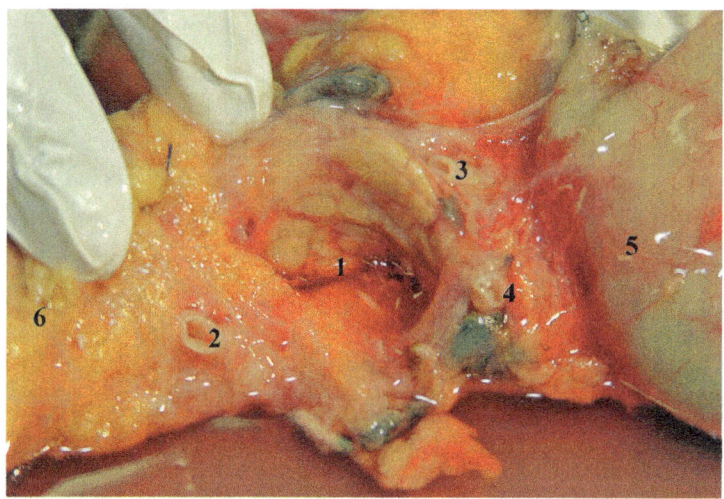

Fig. 15.60 Pancreas procured for islet isolation. 1 – Vena porta has been cut at the level of the SMV and splenic vein, 2 – Short cut splenic artery, 3 – Gastroduodenal artery, 4 – Ligated CBD, 5 – Duodenum, 6 – Pancreas body. In this case vessels have not been marked with polypropylene surgical suture

15.3.5 Summary

- Pancreas capsule must be intact.
- All abnormalities concerning pancreatic ducts have to be recognised, saved and not damaged.
- Spleen hilum should be intact. Common bile duct has to be ligated.
- Pancreatic vessels can be cut short. They are not important during the process of islet isolation
- External cooling of the pancreas with sterile ice during organ procurement has a positive influence on the amount and the viability of isolated of islets of Langerhans (14, 15, 16, 17, 18, 19, 20, 21).

15.4 Liver Procurement

15.4.1 Surgical Steps

1. Cut from IVC patch with the left renal vein, and place it on the left from abdominal aorta (Figs. 15.61 and 15.62).
2. Through the left renal vein opening in the IVC localize the ostium of the right renal vein (s) (Fig. 15.63).

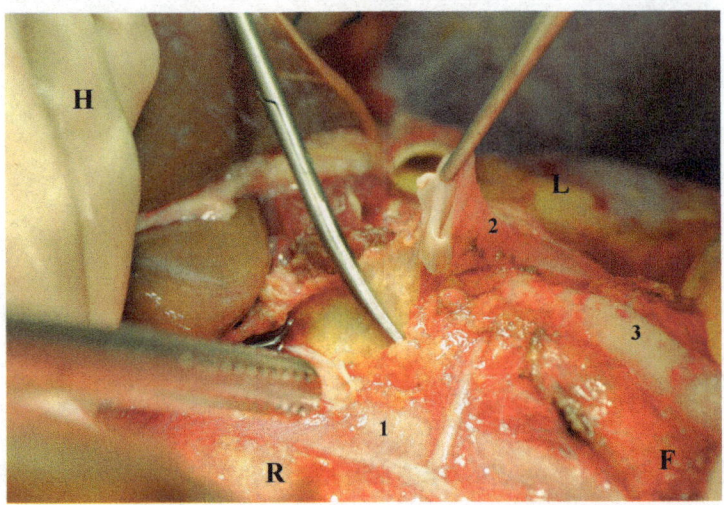

Fig. 15.61 Bisected left renal vein from IVC. 1 – IVC, 2 – left renal vein, 3 – abdominal aorta, *H – head, F – feet, R –right, L – left*

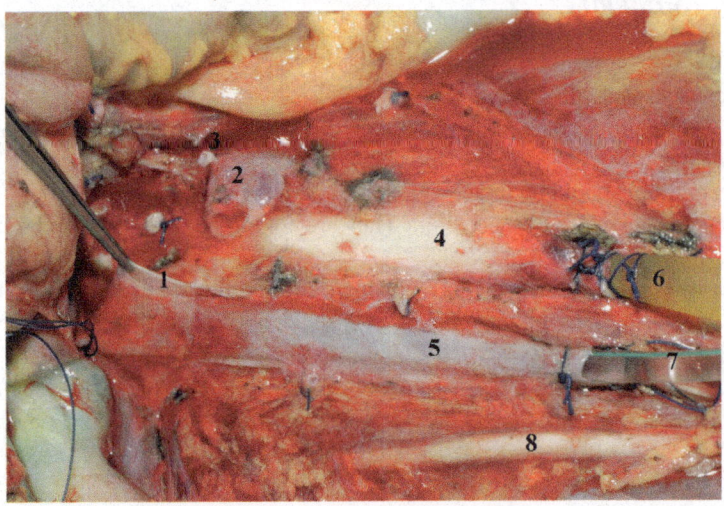

Fig. 15.62 1 – Bisected left renal vein, 2 – Opening in the IVC after cutting the left renal vein, 3 – Ligated left adrenal vein, 4 – Abdominal aorta, 5 – IVC, 6 – Aorta cannula, 7 – IVC decompression cannula, 8 – Right ureter, *H – head, F – feet, R –right, L – left*

15.4 Liver Procurement

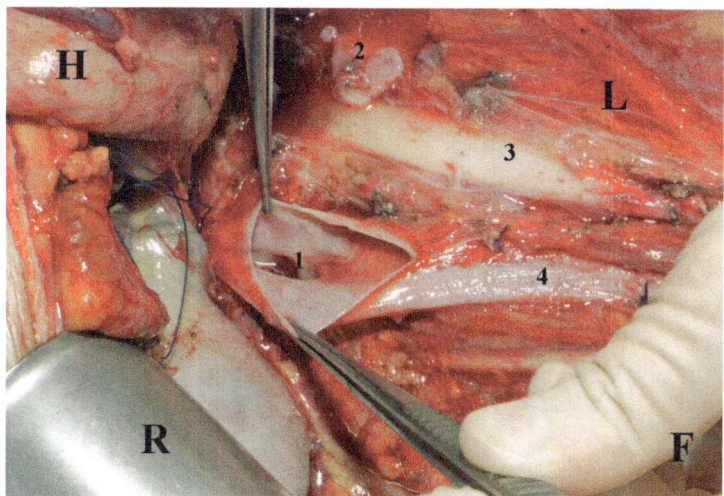

Fig. 15.63 1 – Highest situated ostium of the right renal vein – view through opening in the IVC, 2 – Severed left renal vein, 3 – Aorta, 4 – IVC, *H – head, F – feet, R –right, L – left*

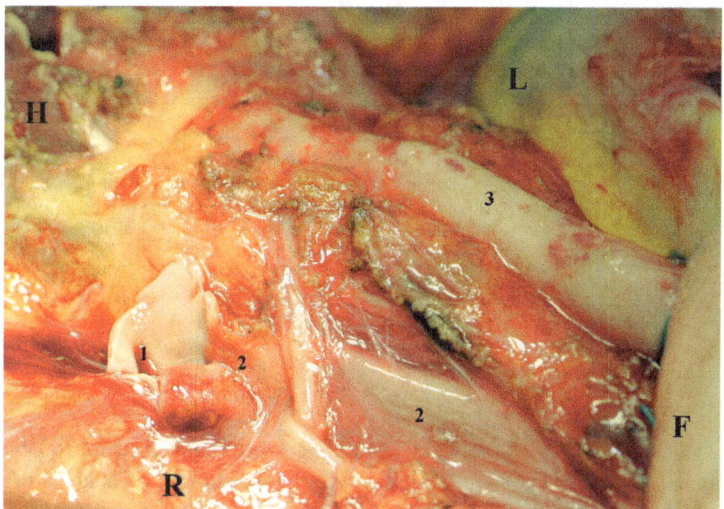

Fig. 15.64 1 – Divided IVC, 2 – IVC, 3 – Abdominal aorta, 4 – Left liver lobe, *H – head, F – feet, R –right, L – left*

3. Cut the IVC below the liver about 1–1.5 cm above the highest situated ostium of the right renal vein (Fig. 15.64).
4. Look at the drawing to see how to divide the IVC between the liver and the right and left kidneys (Fig. 15.65).

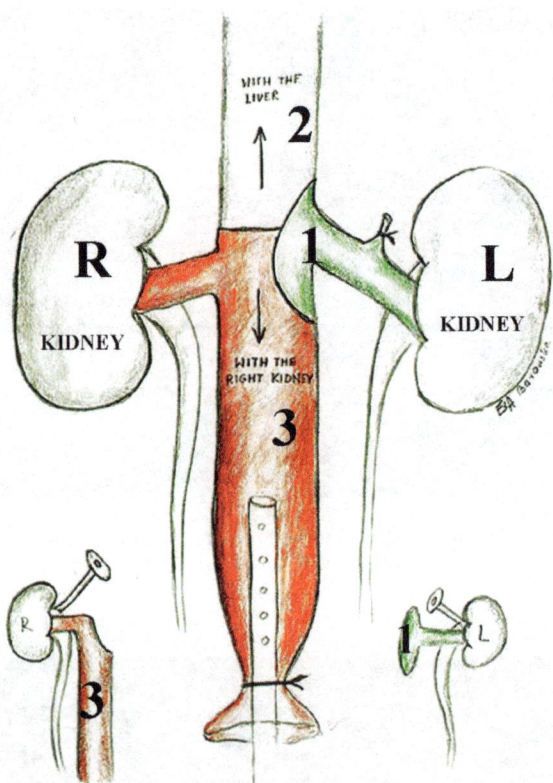

Fig. 15.65 1 – Green part of the IVC has to be given to the left kidney, 2 – White part of the IVC has to be given to the liver, 3 – Red part of the IVC has to be given to the right kidney

5. Cut IVC at the level of the right atrium (if heart is not procured), or ask the thorax surgeon to cut IVC 2–2.5 cm above the diaphragm (if heart is procured) (Fig. 15.66).
6. Put the forefinger in the IVC above the liver and gently hold up the liver during dissection of both leaflets of the diaphragm (Fig. 15.67).
7. Cut left leaflet of the diaphragm. Begin from the left side at the level of the right side of the oesophagus direction, pericardium around the IVC above the diaphragm (Fig. 15.68).
8. Cut the right leaflet of the diaphragm. Pull the liver gently to the left side, cut the right anterior, posterior and lateral part of the diaphragm in the direction downward to the upper pole of the right kidney. Be careful during division of the

15.4 Liver Procurement

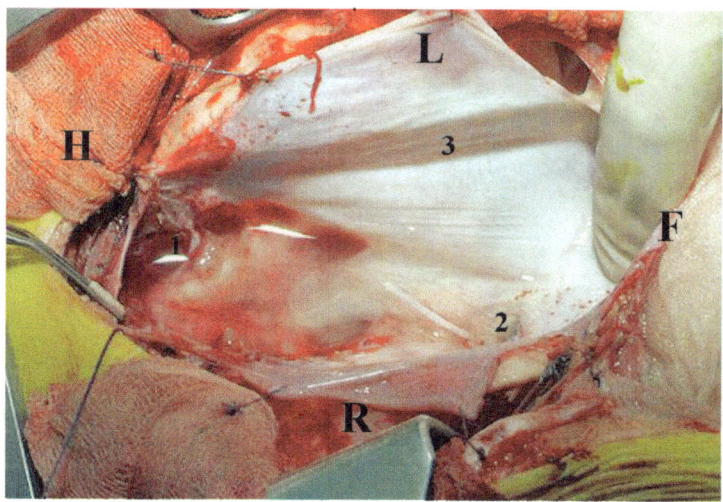

Fig. 15.66 Pericardium after heart procurement. 1 – Bisected superior vena cava, 2 – Bisected IVC above the diaphragm, 3 – Pericardium, *H – head, F – feet, R –right, L – left*

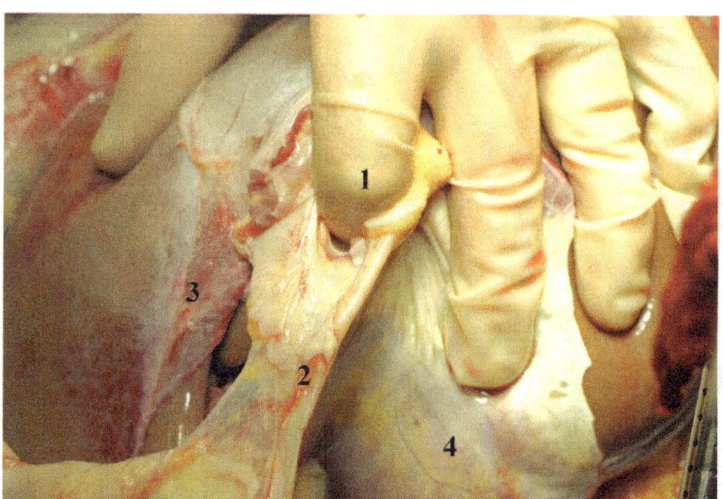

Fig. 15.67 1 – Index finger in the IVC, 2 – Left leaflet of the diaphragm, 3 – Left liver lobe, 4 – Right leaflet of the diaphragm

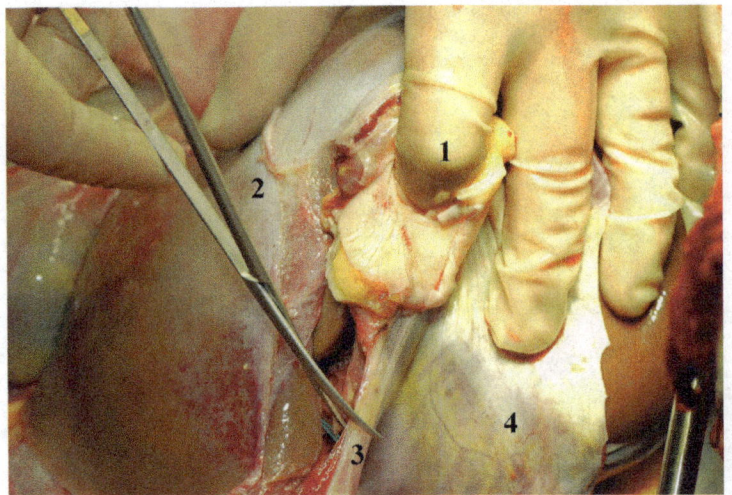

Fig. 15.68 1 – Index finger in the IVC, 2 – Left liver lobe, 3 –Left leaflet of the diaphragm, 4 – Dissected right leaflet of the diaphragm

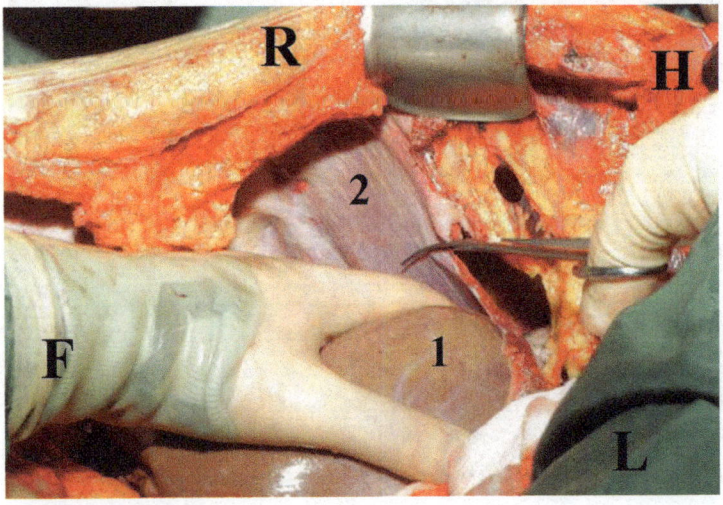

Fig. 15.69 Cutting the right diaphragm. 1 – Right liver lobe, 2 – Right leaflet of the diaphragm, *H – head, F – feet, R –right, L – left*

15.4 Liver Procurement

hepatorenal ligament, stay away from the liver, avoid liver and right kidney capsule and parenchyma injury (Figs. 15.69 and 15.70).

ATTENTION!
- Do not try to dissect the right diaphragm and/or the right adrenal gland from the liver; try to procure the liver with both of them.

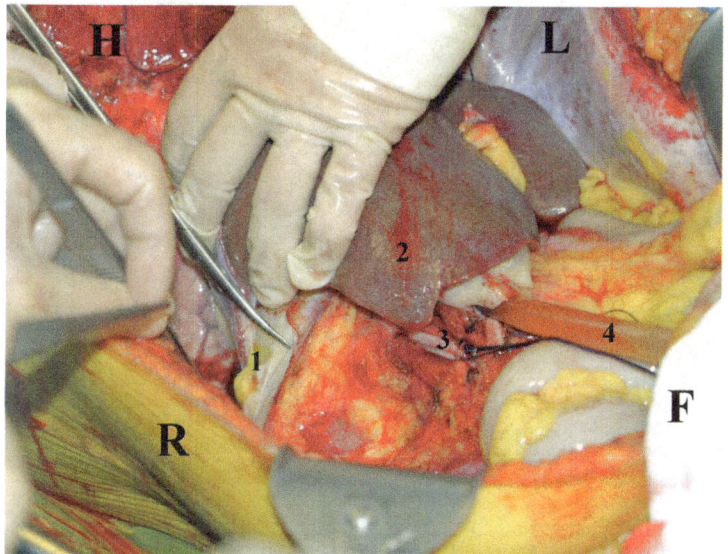

Fig. 15.70 Cutting the right diaphragm. 1 – Posterior part of the right leaflet of the diaphragm, 2 – Right liver lobe, 3 – IVC, 4 – Aorta cannula, *H – head, F – feet, R – right, L – left*

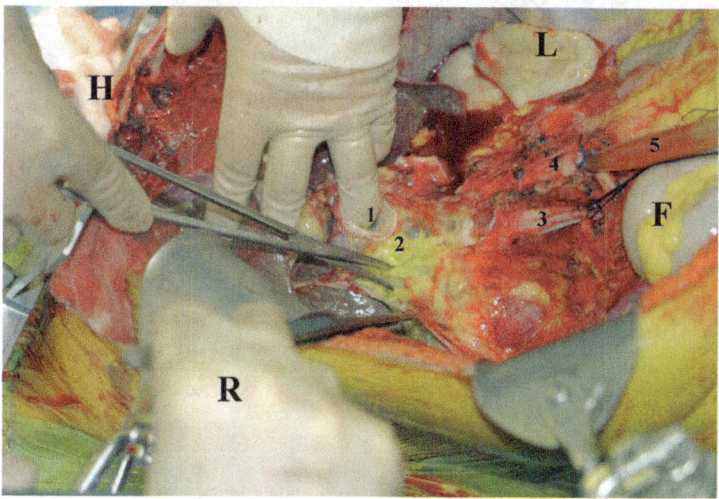

Fig. 15.71 1 – Fourth finger in the IVC, 2 – Dissected retroperitoneal tissues behind IVC, 3 – Distal part of the IVC, 4 – Abdominal aorta, 5 – Aorta cannula, *H – head, F – feet, R – right, L – left*

- Put one finger in the IVC below the liver and gently hold it up and cut the surrounding tissues during final IVC dissection (Figs. 15.71–15.73).
- Place the procured liver in a sterile container filled with ice and cold sterile 0.9% NaCl, Ringer lactate or preservation solution (Fig. 15.74).

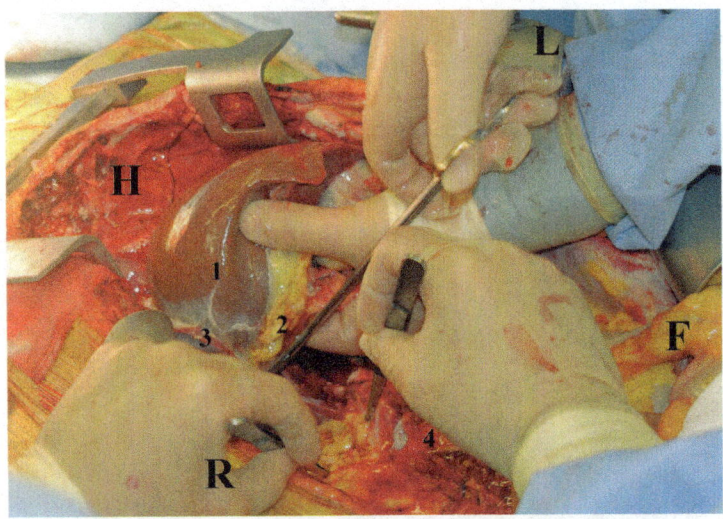

Fig. 15.72 1 – Index finger in the IVC below the liver, 2 – Tissues behind IVC, 3 – Right diaphragm, 4 – IVC, *H – head, F – feet, R –right, L – left*

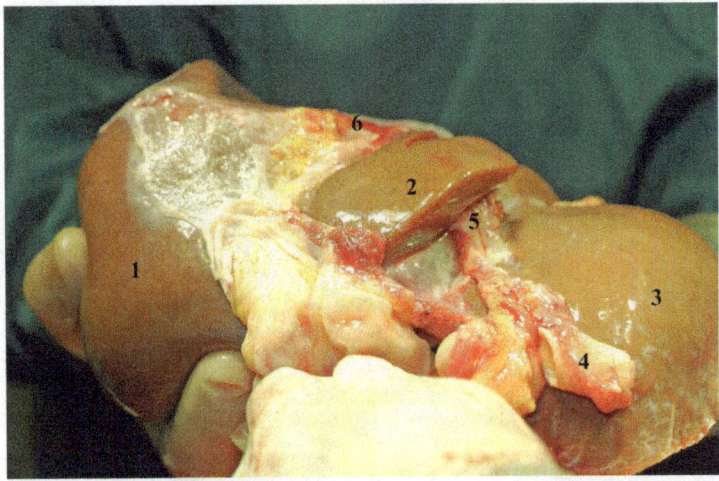

Fig. 15.73 Procured liver. 1 – Right liver lobe, 2 – Caudate lobe, 3 – Left liver lobe, 4 – Celiac trunk with abdominal aorta, 5 – Common hepatic artery, 6 – Hilum of the liver

15.4 Liver Procurement

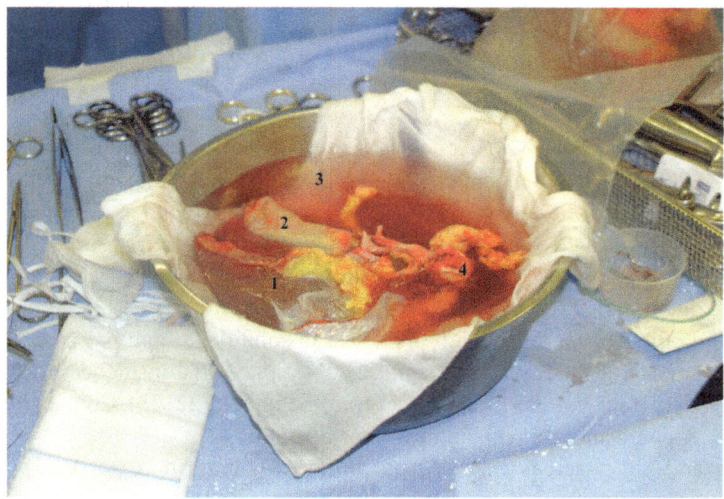

Fig. 15.74 Procured liver, placed in a sterile container filled with sterile ice. 1 – Right liver lobe, 2 – Gallbladder, 3 – Preservation solution, 4 – Abdominal aorta

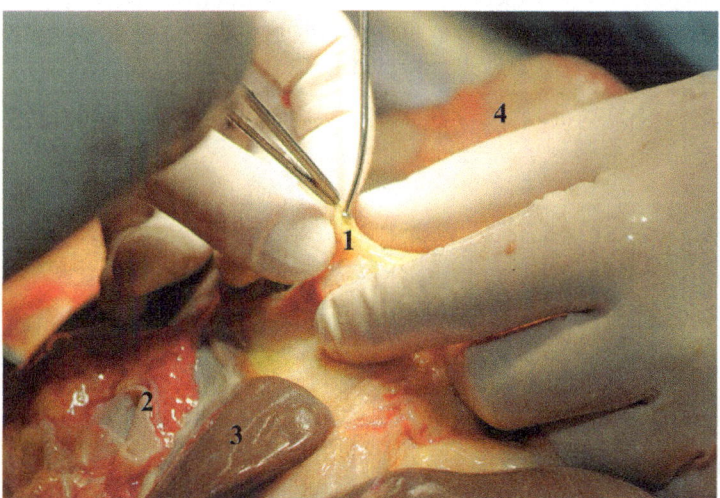

Fig. 15.75 1 – Rinsing the common bile duct and the intra-hepatic biliary tree, 2 – IVC, 3 – Caudate lobe, 4 – Right liver lobe

- Rinse the common bile duct one more time with cold preservation solution (Fig. 15.75).
- If the gallbladder has been not opened and cleaned, ligate the cystic duct or perform cholecystectomy with cystic duct ligation.

- Before packing, perform a liver inspection one more times for state of parenchyma, quality of perfusion, arterial vascularisation, biliary tree and damages during procurement.

ATTENTION
- If the anatomy of the cystic duct or the hepatic artery is not clear, stay away from the liver hilum, and open and clean the gallbladder and the common bile duct.
- It is always better to perform cholecystectomy in the recipient hospital instead of very complicated vascular reconstruction of the hepatic artery, which has been damaged by the donor surgeon during a quick cholecystectomy and/or cystic duct ligation.
- Flushing the hepatic artery with preservation solution at high pressure after the procurement for the back table significantly reduces the incidence of ischemic type biliary tract lesion 3 months after transplantation (22, 23). Contact recipient centre if you want to do this in the donor hospital.
- Liver and the pancreas *en block* procurement – indications (Figs. 15.76 and 15.77) are as follows:

- Standard surgical technique of the procurement centre followed by splitting on the back table in the donor or recipient hospital.
- Unstable donor organ splitting outside the body (back table).
- Abnormal anatomy of the liver – impossible to split liver and the pancreas and make these two organs suitable for transplantation. In most of the cases, the pancreas has to be offered to save the liver.

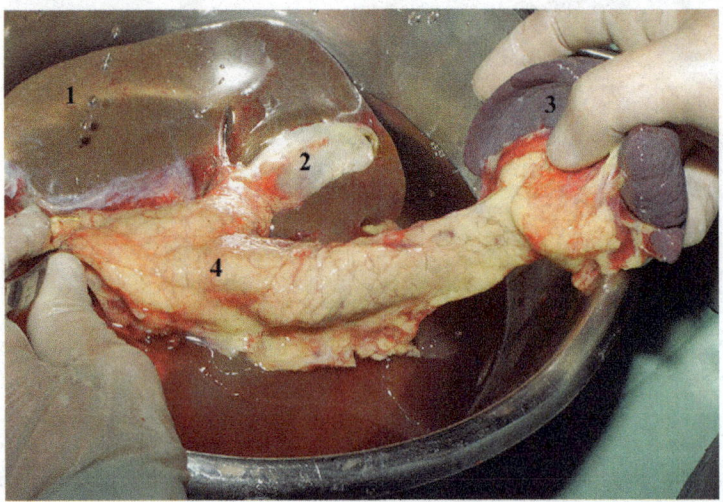

Fig. 15.76 1 – Liver, 2 – Opened and flushed gallbladder, 3 – Spleen, 4 – Pancreas

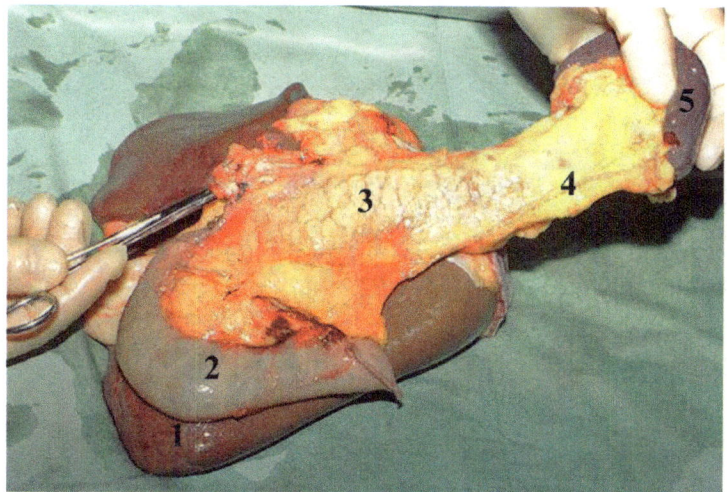

Fig. 15.77 1 – Right liver lobe, 2 – Duodenum, 3 – Pancreas, 4 – Stapler line – transverse mesocolon has been closed and divided, 5 –splenic hilum intact

- Non-heart-beating donor procedure – because of lack of vessel pulsation, it is almost impossible to recognize an arterial abnormality after cardiac death (12).

15.5 Kidney Procurement (24–28)

15.5.1 Separately: Surgical Steps

1. Cut the ligatures placed on the aorta and the IVC (Fig. 15.78).
2. Remove cannulas perfusing the aorta and decompressing the IVC (Fig. 15.79).
3. Open longitudinally anterior wall of the abdominal aorta. Stay exactly in the middle (Fig. 15.80).
4. Check on the ostia of the renal arteries; look for accessory renal artery from aorta or/and from the iliac arteries (Fig. 15.81). If you have any doubts gently use a very thin Fogarthy's catheter or Venflon to localize renal aberrant arteries.
5. Cut off the abdominal aorta above bifurcation and open its posterior wall longitudinally. Stay exactly on the tissues covering vertebral bodies in the middle between lumbar arteries (Fig. 15.82).
6. Cut off inferior vena cava (IVC) above its bifurcation (Fig. 15.83).
7. Mobilise each kidney with pararenal and perirenal fat from retroperitoneum right up to the vertebral column together with the ureter(s) with as much as

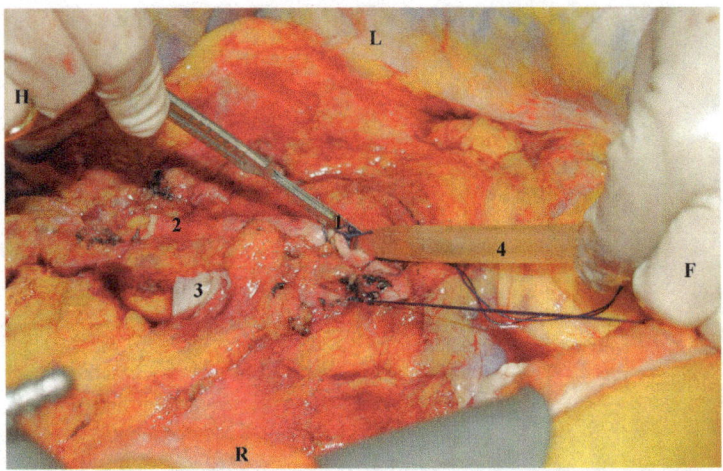

Fig. 15.78 1 – Severing the aortic ligature, 2 – Abdominal aorta, 3 – Bisected IVC below the liver, 4 – Aorta cannula, *H – head, F – feet, R –right, L – left*

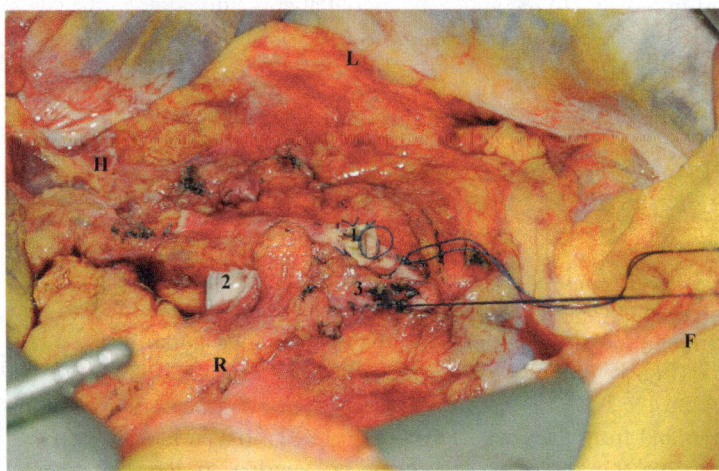

Fig. 15.79 Aorta and IVC cannulas have been removed. 1 – Aorta, 2 – IVC below the liver, 3 – IVC above bifurcation, *H – head, F – feet, R –right, L – left*

15.5 Kidney Procurement

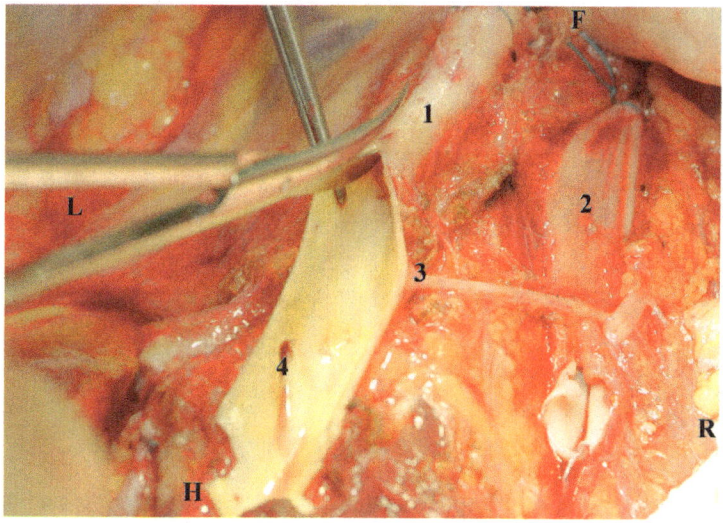

Fig. 15.80 Aorta anterior side opening. 1 – Aorta close to the bifurcation, 2 – IVC, 3 – Right aberrant renal artery, 4 – Left renal artery, *H – head, F – feet, R –right, L – left*

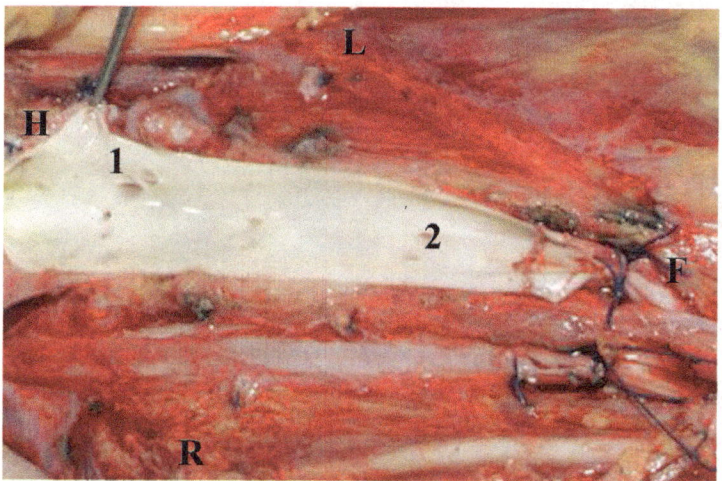

Fig. 15.81 1 – Ostia of the two left renal arteries, 2 – Lumbar artery, *H – head, F – feet, R –right, L – left*

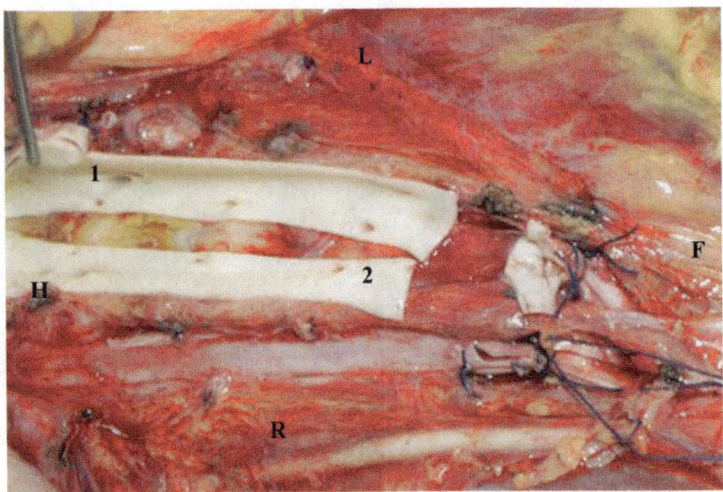

Fig. 15.82 Aorta bisected above her bifurcation. Splitting the posterior wall of the abdominal aorta between lumbar arteries. 1 – Ostia of the left two renal arteries, 2 – Aorta patch of the right kidney with lumbar arteries, *H – head, F – feet, R – right, L – left*

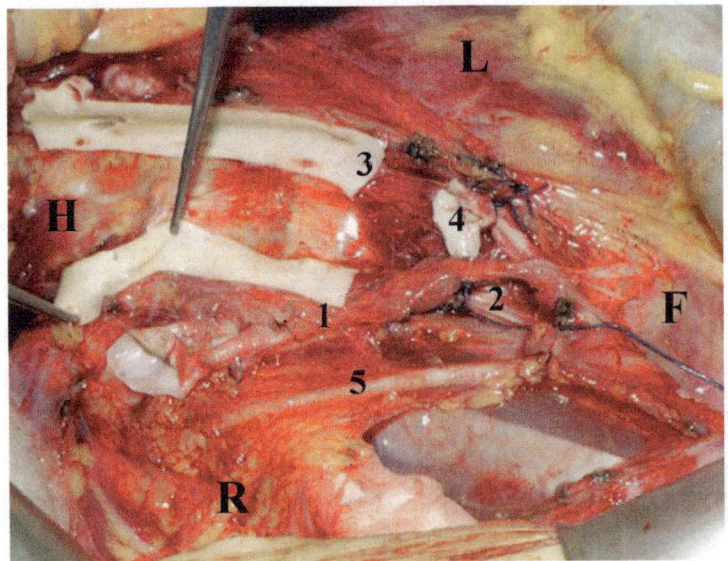

Fig. 15.83 1 – IVC cut off above bifurcation, 2 – Bifurcation of IVC, 3 – Abdominal aorta bisected above bifurcation, 4 – Aorta cut off at the bifurcation, 5 – Right ureter, *H – head, F – feet, R – right, L – left*

possible adjacent tissue as far down towards the urinary bladder as possible (Figs. 15.84 and 15.85).
8. Holding and lifting gently each kidney in your hand. Mobilise with scissors left and right aorta patches and the IVC (the right kidney) from the tissues covering vertebral bodies (Figs. 15.86 and 15.87).

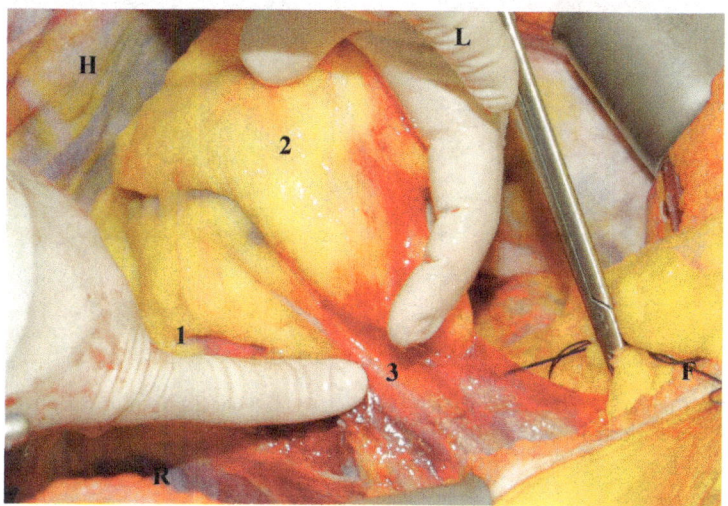

Fig. 15.84 Kidney mobilisation. 1 – Retroperitoneum, 2 – Mobilised right kidney from the retroperitoneum, 3 – Ureter, *H – head, F – feet, R –right, L – left*

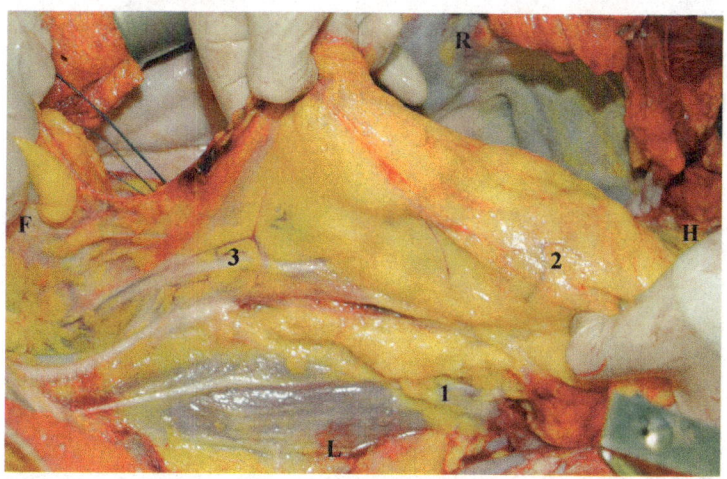

Fig. 15.85 Kidney mobilisation. 1 – Retroperitoneum, 2 – Mobilised left kidney from retroperitoneum, 3 – Ureter, *H – head, F – feet, R –right, L – left*

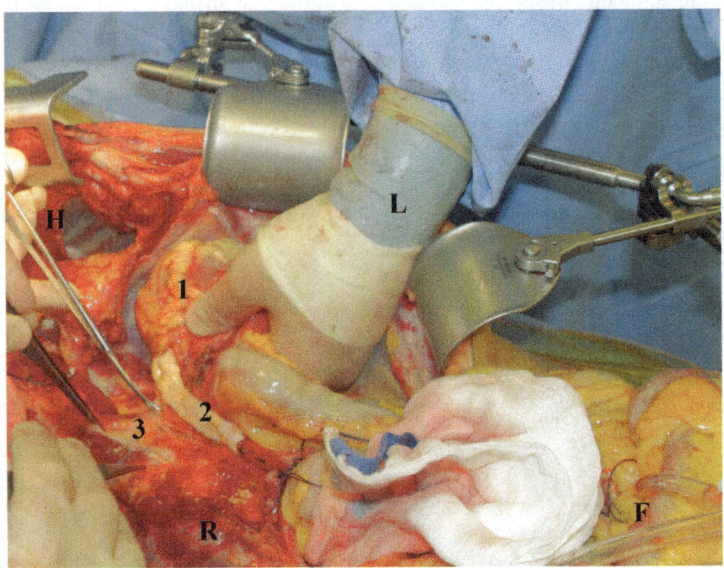

Fig. 15.86 Cutting aortic patch for the left kidney. 1 – Left kidney, 2 – Aortic patch with ostium of the left renal artery, 3 – Vertebral column, *H – head, F – feet, R –right, L – left*

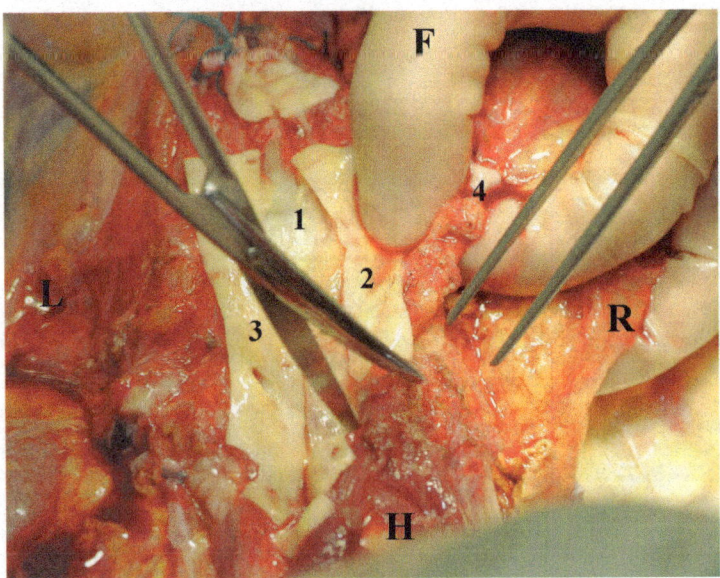

Fig. 15.87 Mobilising the right and the left kidney aorta patch. 1 – Vertebral column, 2 – Right aorta patch, 3 – Left aorta patch, 4 – IVC, *H – head, F – feet, R –right, L – left*

15.5 Kidney Procurement

9. Cut the ureters close to the urinary bladder (Figs. 15.88 and 15.89).
10. Take out each kidney separately and place in a sterile container filled with ice and cold sterile 0.9% NaCl or Ringer lactate or preservation solution (Fig. 15.90).

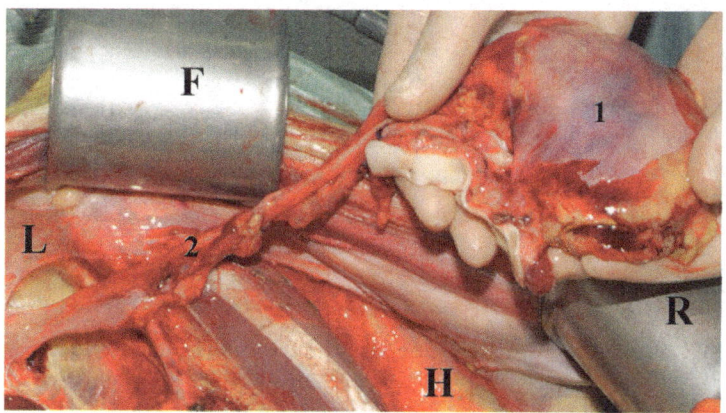

Fig. 15.88 1 – Kidney, 2 – Ureter with surrounding tissues, *H – head, F – feet, R –right, L – left*

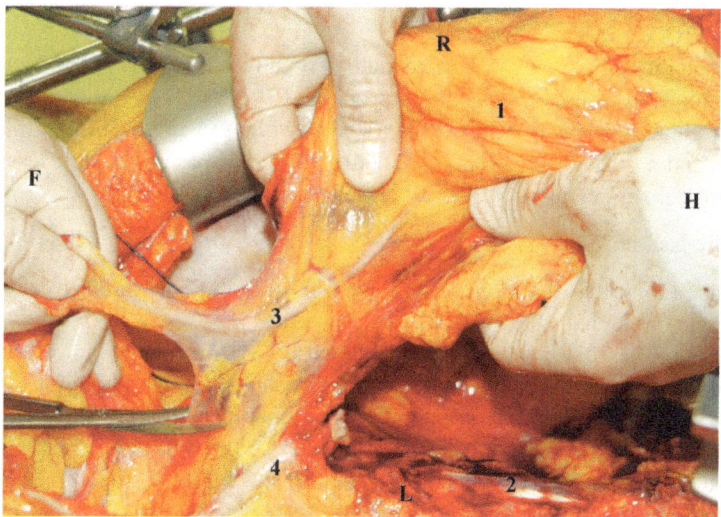

Fig. 15.89 1 – Mobilised left kidney, 2 – Retroperitoneum, 3 –Bisected ureter, 4 – Left common iliac artery, *H – head, F – feet, R –right, L – left*

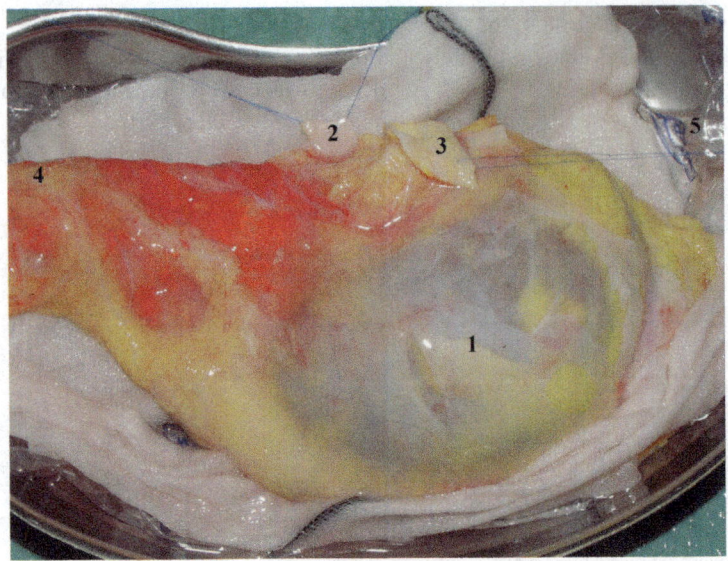

Fig. 15.90 Left kidney placed in a sterile container filled with sterile Ringer solution and ice. 1 – Kidney with para- and perirenal fat – anterior side small amount 2 – Left renal vein, 3 – Renal artery with aortic patch, 4 – Ureter

ATTENTION!
- Left and the right kidney should be loudly (vocally) indicated and marked on the table to avoid mistakes during organ packing (Fig. 15.91).
- The right kidney has to be procured together with IVC, in case of multiple renal veins and a difficult recipient. IVC could be of use, of course, if necessary for right renal vein elongation (Fig. 15.92).

Before packing:

- Reduce fat around the kidney. Stay away from the kidney hilum (renal artery, vein and the ureter) (Fig. 15.93).
- Leave sufficient tissues around the ureters (do not strip them) (Fig. 15.94).
- Examine each kidney (Figs. 15.95 and 15.96) and the ureter(s), paying attention to the following: presence of a tumour or an injury, state of perfusion (if inadequate try to reperfuse before packing), vascular anatomy, state of arteriosclerosis of the renal arteries and the abdominal aorta, checking for signs of an infected cyst, polycystic disease or ureter stenosis.
- If necessary perform biopsy and inform acceptor centre(s) about your findings of inclusive organ transplantability.

15.5 Kidney Procurement

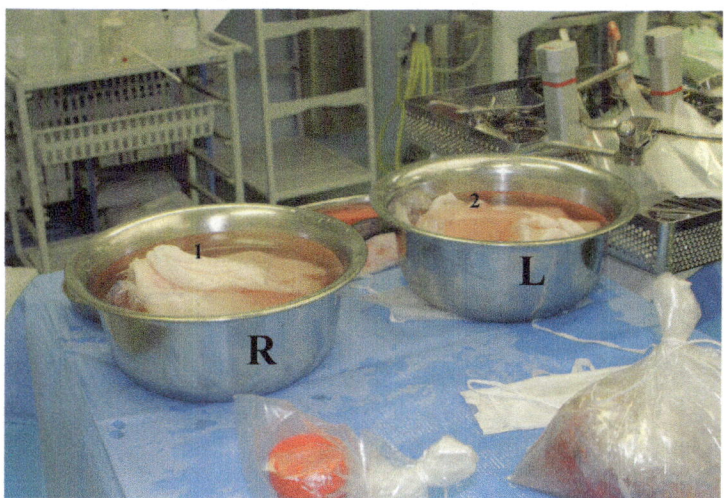

Fig. 15.91 R – Right container for the right kidney, L – Left container for the left kidney – this must be clear to avoid mistakes during organ packing. 1 – Right kidney, 2 – Left kidney

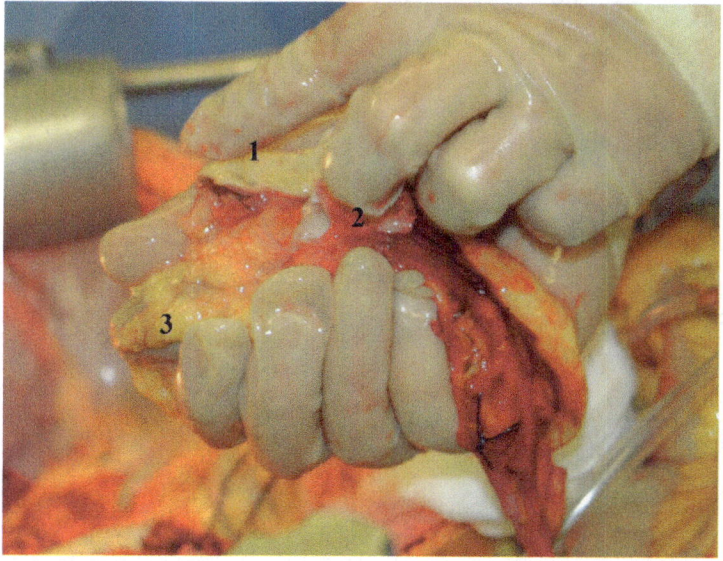

Fig. 15.92 Procured right kidney. 1 – Renal artery with aortic patch, 2 – IVC, 3 – Upper pole

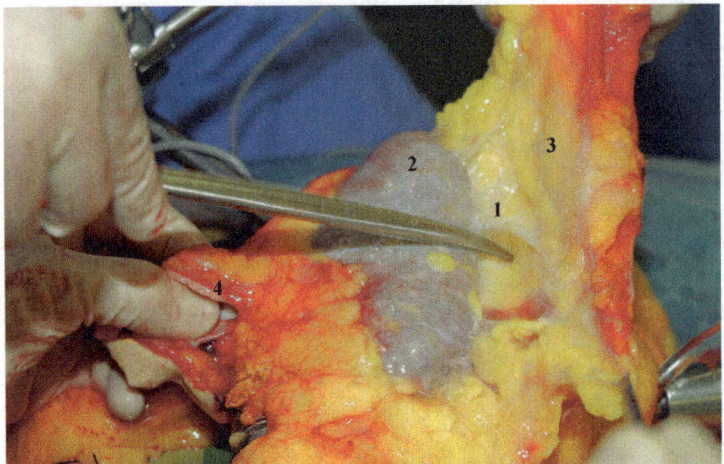

Fig. 15.93 1 – Perirenal fat, 2 – Kidney, 3 – Pararenal fat abundant on the posterior kidney side, 4 – Renal vessels

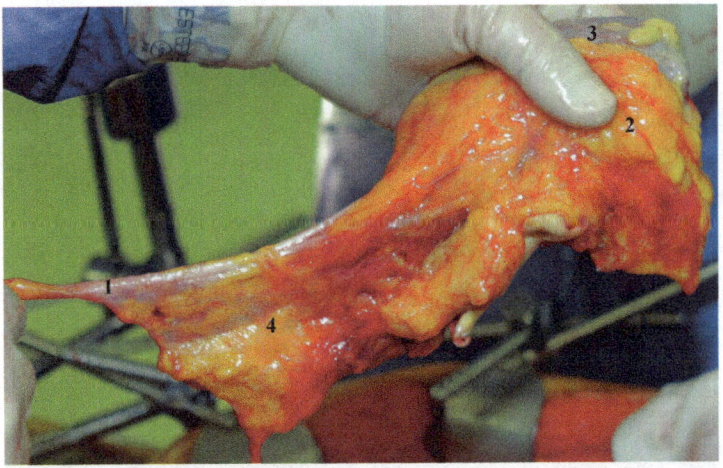

Fig. 15.94 1 – Long ureter, 2 – Pararenal fat, 3 – Kidney, 4 – Retroperitoneal tissues surrounding the ureter

15.5.2 En Block Kidney Procurement: Surgical Steps

1. Mobilise both kidneys from retro-peritoneum.
2. Cut the ligatures placed on the aorta and the IVC (Fig. 15.97).
3. Remove the cannulas perfusing the aorta and decompressing the IVC (Fig. 15.98).

15.5 Kidney Procurement

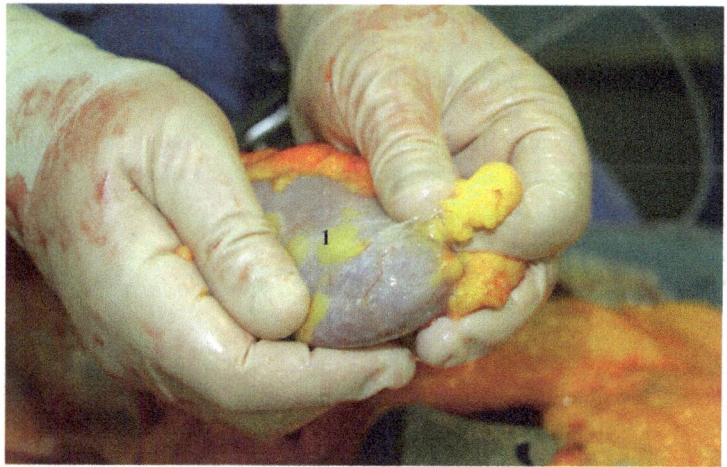

Fig. 15.95 Kidney examination. 1 – Kidney surface

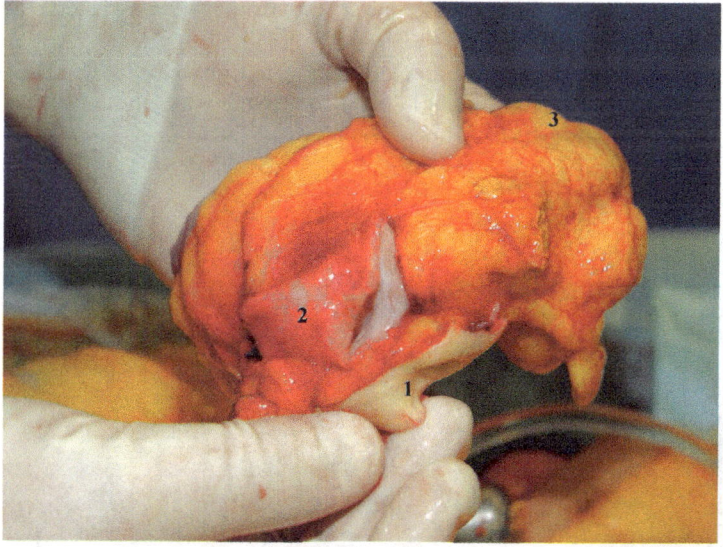

Fig. 15.96 Examination of the renal vessels. 1 – Aorta patch with ostium of the renal artery, 2 – Renal vein, 3 – Perirenal fat

4. Mobilise and cut aorta, IVC above their bifurcations and the ureters close to the urinary bladder. With a small mosquito clamp, close their walls, via lumen together and gently lift them up (Fig. 15.99).

5. Cut all the tissues passing posterior to the aorta and IVC close to the vertebral ligaments and the muscles covering the vertebral bodies (Fig. 15.100). Cut the tissues going upwards until the previous trans-sections of aorta and IVC are reached.
6. Take out the kidneys and place them in a cooled preservation solution bath with ice and if necessary separated on the back table (Fig. 15.101).

15.5.3 Separation of Kidneys Procured En Block in Steps

1. Introduction
2. Surgical technique of separation of kidneys retrieved en block on the back table is almost the same as separation in situ, with only one difference that you have to begin on the back table with the aorta posterior wall incision (look at Sect. 15.2.1).
3. Mark and recognize on both sides the number and the position of the ureters.
4. Incise longitudinally the posterior wall of the abdominal aorta between the lumbar arteries.
5. Check the number of renal arteries arising from abdominal aorta for each kidney.
6. Turn the kidneys over; remove the left renal vein from the VCI with a patch.
7. Incise the anterior wall of the abdominal aorta. Stay correctly in the mid-line.
8. Before packing:

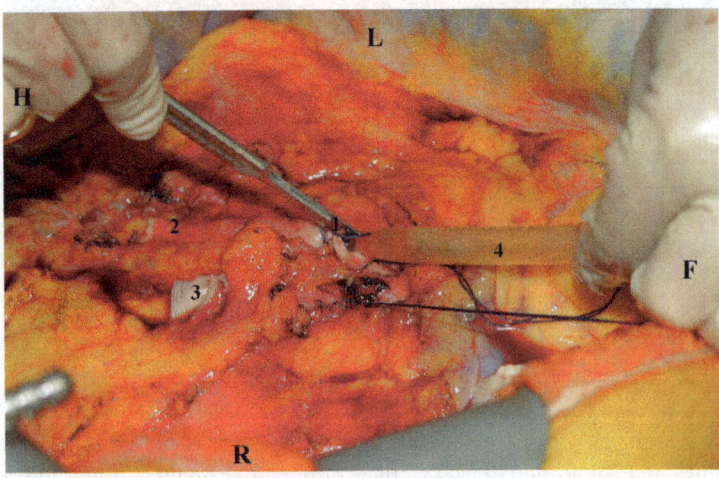

Fig. 15.97 1 – Cutting off the aortic ligature, 2 – Abdominal aorta, 3 – Cut IVC below the liver, 4 – Aorta cannula, *H – head, F – feet, R –right, L – left*

15.5 Kidney Procurement

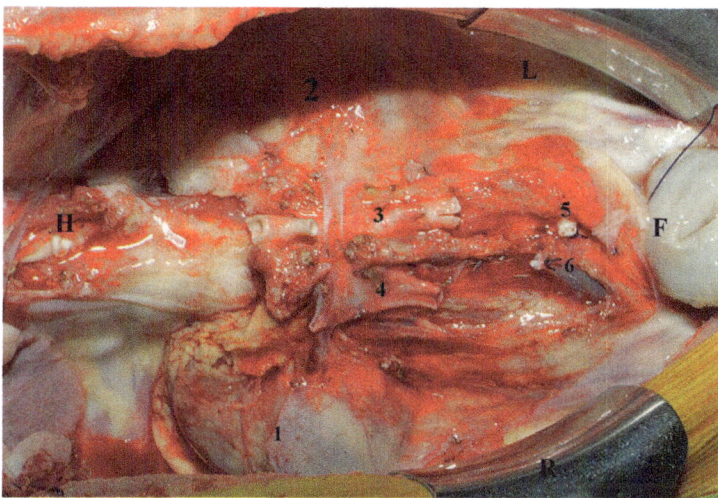

Fig. 15.98 Aorta and IVC cannulas have been removed. 1 – Right kidney, 2 – Left kidney, 3 – Aorta, 4 – IVC, 5 – Aortic bifurcation, 6 – IVC bifurcation, *H – head, F – feet, R – right, L – left*

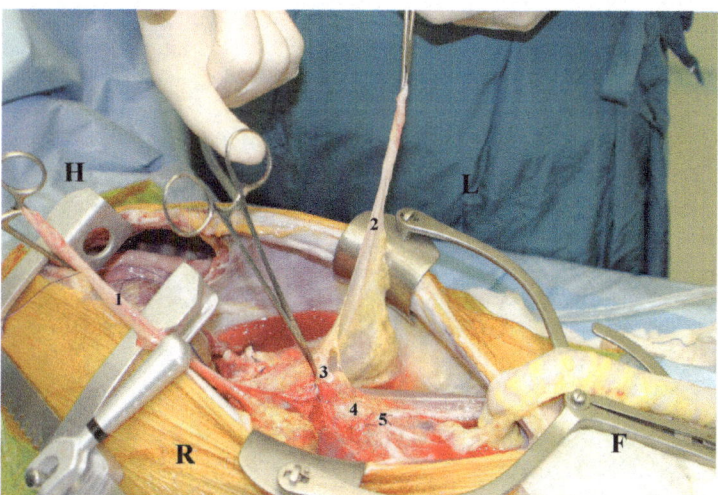

Fig. 15.99 1 – Right ureter, 2 – Left ureter, 3 – Vertebral column, 4 – Aorta and IVC clamp together with mosquito clamp, 5 – Bifurcations of the aorta and IVC, *H – head, F – feet, R – right, L – left*

- Reduce the fat around the kidney and the ureter.
- During fat reduction, stay away from the kidney hilum, tissues around the ureters and away from the vessels.

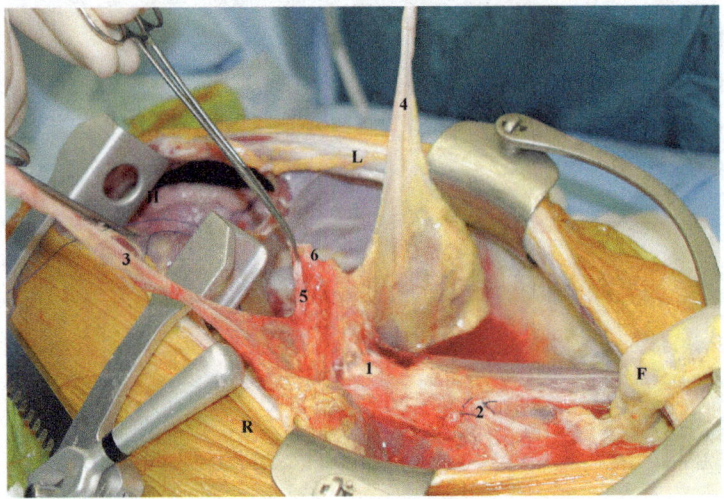

Fig. 15.100 1 – Tissues covering vertebral bodies, 2 – Aorta and IVC bifurcations, 3 – Right ureter, 4 – Left ureter, 5 – IVC, 6 – Aorta, *H – head, F – feet, R –right, L – left*

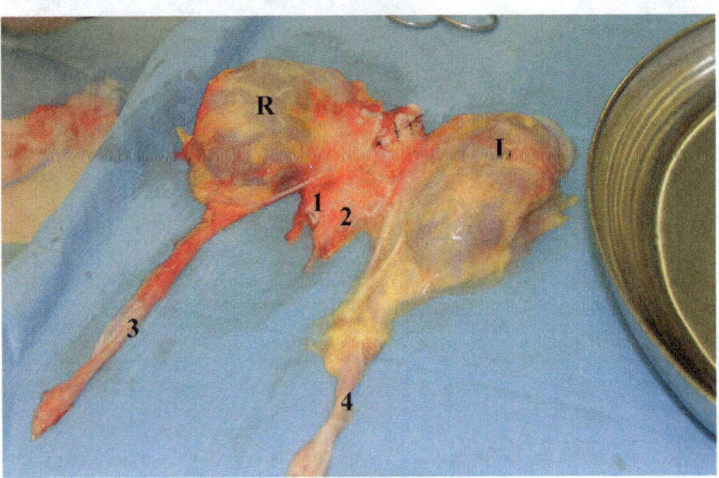

Fig. 15.101 Kidneys procured en block. R – Right kidney, L – Left kidney, 1 – IVC, 2 – Abdominal aorta, 3 – Right ureter, 4 – Left ureter

- Examine each kidney and the ureter one more time for checking the following: state of perfusion (very important – if bad, reperfuse before packing), vascular anatomy, state of arteriosclerosis, renal arteries and abdominal aorta for tumour, injury, infection, cyst, polycystic disease and ureter stenosis.

- If necessary perform biopsy and inform acceptor centre(s) about your findings of inclusive organ transplantability.

ATTENTION!
- The detailed dissection of the kidney structures should be left to the transplant surgeon from the recipient centre.
- In case of poor kidney perfusion or uncertainty as to whether there are pre-existing diseases, a biopsy should be performed and evaluated by the pathologist of the recipient centre (inform the transplant coordinator and the recipient(s) centre(s) about your findings).
- In the case of donors ≤ 5 years, both kidneys should be removed en bloc, including complete abdominal aorta and IVC – from their bifurcations up to SMA and 1 cm above the renal veins (IVC).
- When faced with child donors, always discuss your kidney procurement technique with kidney(s) acceptor centre(s) (Fig. 15.101).

Literature

1. Starzl TE, Miller C, Broznick B, Makowka L (1987) An improved technique for multiple organ harvesting. Surg Gynecol Obstet: 165: 343-348
2. Yersiz H, Renz JF, Hisatake GM et al (2003) Multivisceral and isolated intestinal procurement techniques. Liver Transpl: 9(8): 881-886
3. Nghiem DD, Schulak JA, Corry RJ (1987) Duodenopancreatectomy for transplantation. Arch Surg: 122: 1201-1206
4. Boggi U, Vistoli F, Del Chiaro M et al (2004) A simplified technique for the en bloc procurement of abdominal organs that is suitable for pancreas and small-bowel transplantation. Surgery: 1(35): 629-641
5. Rosenthal JT, Shaw BJ Jr, Hardesty RL et al (1983) Principles of multiple organ procurement from cadaver donors. Ann Surg: 198: 617-621
6. Casavilla A, Selby R, Abu-Elmagd K et al (1992) Logistics and technique for combined hepatic-intestinal retrieval. Ann Surg: 216: 605-609
7. Sindhi R, Fox IJ, Heffron T et al (1995) Procurement and preparation of human isolated small intestinal grafts for transplantation. Transplantation: 60: 771-773
8. Marsh CL, Perkins JD, Sutherland DER et al (1989) Combined hepatic and pancreaticoduodenal procurement for transplantation. Surg Gynecol Obstet: 168: 254-258
9. Jeon H, Ortiz JA, Manzarbeitia CY, Alvarez SC et al (2002) Combined liver and pancreas procurement from a controlled non-heart-beating donor with aberrant hepatic arterial anatomy. Transplantation: 74: 1636-1639
10. Sollinger HW, Vernon WB, D'Alessandro AM et al (1989) Combined liver and pancreas procurement with Belzer-UW solution. Surgery: 106: 685-690
11. Shaffer D, Lewis WD, Jenkins RL, et al (1992) Combined liver and whole pancreas procurement in donors with a replaced right hepatic artery. Surg Gynecol Obstet: 175: 204-207
12. Mizrahi SS, Jones JW, Bentley FR (1996) Preparing for pancreas transplantation: donor selection, retrieval technique, preservation, and back-table preparation. Transpl Rev: 10: 1-12
13. Stratta RJ, Taylor RJ, Spees EK et al (1991) Refinements in cadaveric pancreas-kidney procurement and preservation. Transpl Proc: 23: 2320-2322
14. Nagata H, Matsumoto S, Okitsu T et al (2006) Procurement of the human pancreas for pancreatic islet transplantation from marginal cadaver donors. Transplantation: 82(3): 327-333

15. Frutos MA, Ruiz P, Mansilla JJ (2005) Pancreas donation for islet transplantation. Transpl Proc: 37(3): 1560-1561
16. Truong W, Lakey JR, Ryan EA, Shapiro AM (2005) Clinical islet transplantation at the University of Alberta–the Edmonton experience. Clin Transpl: 153–172
17. Nagata H, Matsumoto S, Okitsu T (2005) In situ cooling of pancreata from non-heart-beating donors prior to procurement for islet transplantation. Transpl Proc: 37(8): 3393-3395
18. Lee TC, Barshes NR, Brunicardi FC (2004) Procurement of the human pancreas for pancreatic islet transplantation. Transplantation: 78(3): 481-483
19. Nagata H, Matsumoto S, Okitsu T, Iwanaga Y (2006) Procurement of the human pancreas for pancreatic islet transplantation from marginal cadaver donors. Transplantation: 82(3): 327-331
20. Caballero-Corbalan J, Eich T et al (2007) No beneficial effect of two-layer storage compared with uw-storage on human islet isolation and transplantation. Transplantation: 84(7): 864-869
21. Lakey JR, Kneteman NM, Rajotte RV (2002) Effect of core pancreas temperature during cadaveric procurement on human islet isolation and functional viability. Transplantation: 73(7): 1106-1110
22. Moench C, Moench K, Lohse AW et al (2003) Prevention of ischemic type biliary lesions by arterial back-table pressure perfusion. Liver Transpl: 9: 285-289
23. Blumhardt G, Lemmens P, Topalidis T et al (1993) Increased flow rate of preservation solution in the hepatic artery during organ preservation can improve postischemic liver function. Transpl Proc: 25: 2540-2542
24. Ackermann JR, Snell ME (1968) Cadaveric renal transplantation: a technique for donor kidney removal. Br J Urol: 40: 515-521
25. Amante AJ, Kahan BD (1996) En bloc transplantation of kidneys from pediatric donors. J Urol: 155: 852-857
26. Baranski AG, Kramer WLM (2007) Chirurgische technieken voor het uitnemen van de abdominale organen bij pediatrische donoren. Handboek Kindertraumatologie Hoofdstuk 18: 199-214, De Tijdstroom (in Dutch)
27. Colberg JE (1980) En bloc excision for cadaver kidneys for transplantation. Arch Surg: 115: 1238-1241
28. Van der Werf WJ, D'Alessandro AM, Hoffmann RM, Knechtle SJ (1998) Procurement, preservation, and transport of cadaver kidneys. Surg Clin North Am: 78: 41-54

Chapter 16
The Toolkit

Abstract Background: The toolkit plays a very important role during organ harvesting and transplantation. It consists of the arteries and the veins removed during organ procurement. The toolkit is used for the reconstruction of different vessels for both the retrieved organ as well as for the vessels of the recipient. The quality of the procured toolkit is very important and has a great influence on organ and recipient survival.

The most popular toolkit comprises the iliac vessels, which consists of common, external and internal artery and the vein. If the iliac toolkit is of a poor quality, the procurement team should look for other vessels such as the aorta, femoral, or even vessels in the limbs.

In most of the cases, the toolkit is given to the liver, pancreas, small bowel and, if necessary, to the kidney if the recipient centre made such a request or if, during procurement, the kidney vessels were damaged.

Conclusion: The quality of the procured toolkit is very important and has a great influence on organ and recipient survival.

Keywords Toolkit Procurement, Vessels, Veins, Arteries

16.1 Important Tool During the Transplantation Process

16.1.1 Composition

1. The most popular *toolkit* is composed of the iliac veins and the arteries (the common iliac artery and vein, the internal iliac artery and vein, and/or the external iliac artery and vein – all of these should be as long as possible) (Fig. 16.1).
2. Other arteries and the veins that can be retrieved and used during transplantation as a toolkit are as follows:
   - Subclavian artery and vein
   - Brachial, radial, ulnar arteries, cephalic and basilic veins

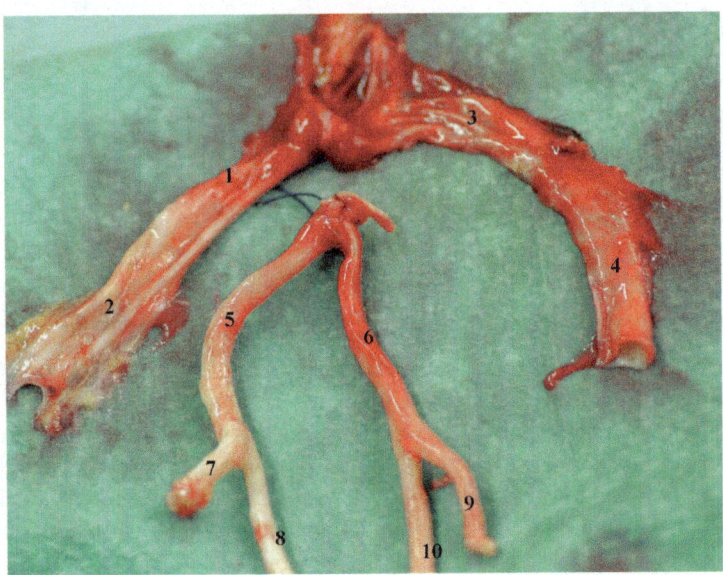

Fig. 16.1 Properly procured toolkit, which consists of arteries and veins. 1 – Right common iliac vein, 2 – Right external iliac vein, 3 – Left common iliac vein, 4 – Left external iliac vein, 5 – Right common iliac artery, 6 – Right common iliac artery, 7 – Right internal iliac artery, 8 – Right external iliac artery, 9 – Left internal iliac artery, 10 – Left external iliac artery

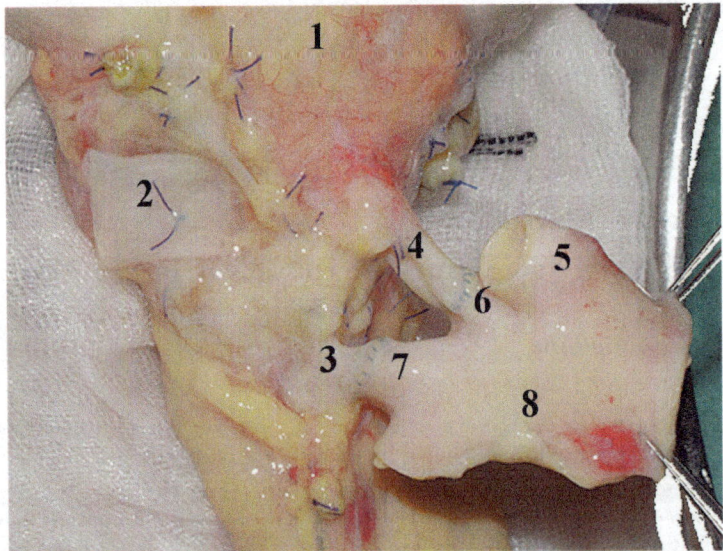

Fig. 16.2 Pancreas arterial reconstruction with the aortic arch. 1 – Pancreas head, 2 – Portal vein, 3 – Splenic artery, 4 – SMA, 5 – Brachycephalic trunk, 6 – Left carotis communis artery, 7 – Left subclavian artery, 8 – Aortic arch wall

16.1 Important Tool During the Transplantation Process

- Arch of the aorta and superior vena cava
- Common internal and external carotid artery and vein
- Femoral artery and the great saphenous vein
- Brachiocephalic artery and vein (Fig. 16.2)

3. Make sure that you are fully informed about the vascular reconstruction, which will be done during back-table or during transplantation in the acceptor centre; this information will help you to choose the most suitable vessels.

16.1.2 Surgical Technique of Toolkit Procurement and Packing

1. Before retrieval, examine the state of the toolkit.
2. In the case of dubious quality, try to find other vessels.
3. Very gently dissect and cut vessels ensuring that they are as long as possible (Fig. 16.3).

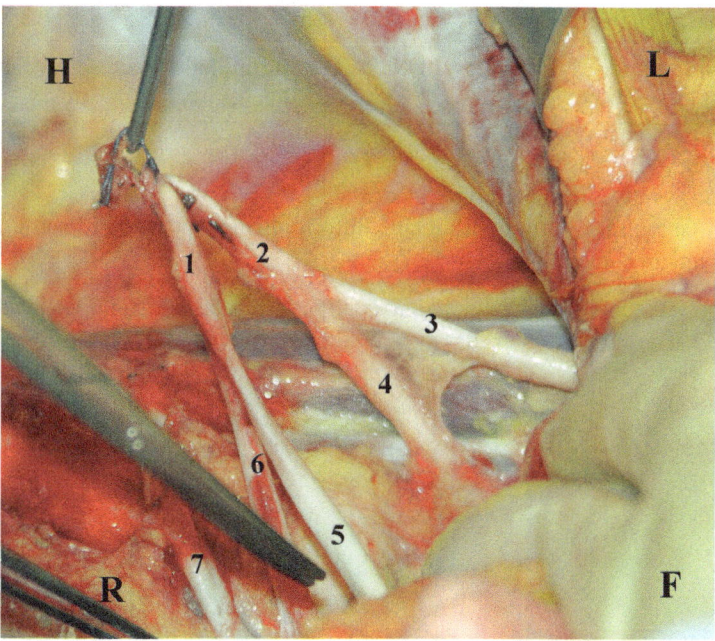

Fig. 16.3 Toolkit procurement – iliac arteries. 1 – Right common iliac artery, 2 – Left common iliac artery, 3 – Left external iliac artery, 4 – Left internal iliac artery, 5 – Right external iliac artery, 6 – Right internal iliac artery, 7 – Right common iliac vein

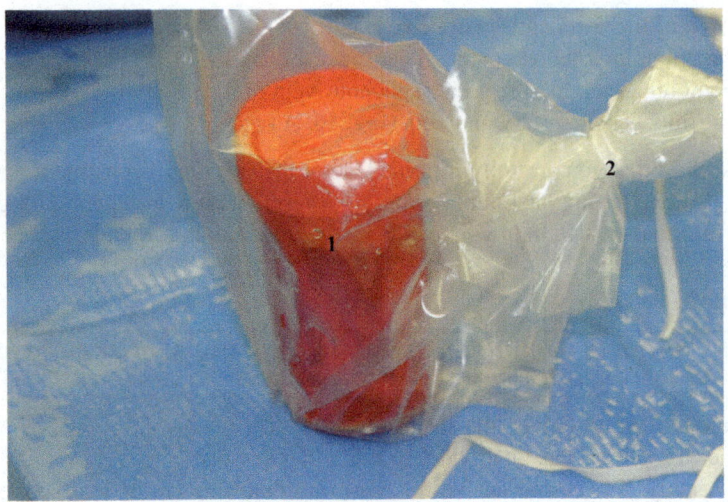

Fig. 16.4 Toolkit packed in sterile container filled with preservation solution and covered with two sterile bags

ATTENTION!
- During artery excision, avoid wall damage, intima dissection and interruption, save small branches and cut them as long as possible or ligate.
- During vein excision avoid the wall damage, save small branches and cut them as long as possible from the main vessel or ligate.
- Always take the best quality toolkit.
- If the toolkit is of dubious quality, inform the transplant coordinator and the recipient centre.

4. If you still have any doubts about quality, try to answer following question: Would I use these vessels myself for organ reconstruction in a young recipient?
5. The toolkit has to be packed according to the same rules as organ packing – see Chap. 17 (Fig. 16.4).

Chapter 17
Organ Packing

Abstract Background: Every organ and the *tool-kit* coming from organ procurement have to be packed according to the Eurotransplant or National Transplant Organization regulations.

The packed organs are placed in an icebox and fully covered with non-sterile, melting ice. Correct packing, without air around every organ, allows good cooling, an optimal temperature during organ transportation and finally good preservation.

Another method of organ preservation and transportation is Kravitz's LifePort Kidney Transporter (Organ recovery), organ preservation and recovery system. The first kidney perfused during transportation by LifePort was transplanted in 2003.

Conclusion: Organ packing following international or national rules plays an important role in the whole process of organ procurement and transplantation, and it can have a very big influence of both organ and patient survival.

Keywords Organ packing, Organ transportation, Transport box, Organ recovery

17.1 Technique of Organ Packing

17.1.1 Introduction

All procured abdominal organs have to be packed according to the Eurotransplant or National Transplant Organization regulations. According to the Eurotransplant regulations each organ is stored in three separate bags, covered with ice in a transport box.

17.1.2 Organ Packing in Steps

- The first bag is filled with a cold preservation solution. The procured organ must be completely covered by the preservation solution, and the bag must be closed (well tied) without any air (Fig. 17.1).
- The second bag (or a wax-impregnated fibre container) is filled with cooled saline or Ringer lactate solution. The first tied bag must be completely covered in one of the solutions and closed (well tied) without air (Fig. 17.2).
- It is recommended to keep the third bag dry, without air, well tied and sometimes covered with a sterile drape (Figs. 17.3 and 17.4).
- Finally the organ is placed is an icebox and well covered with non-sterile melting ice (Fig. 17.5); the box is firmly closed and the organ is ready for transportation (Fig. 17.6).

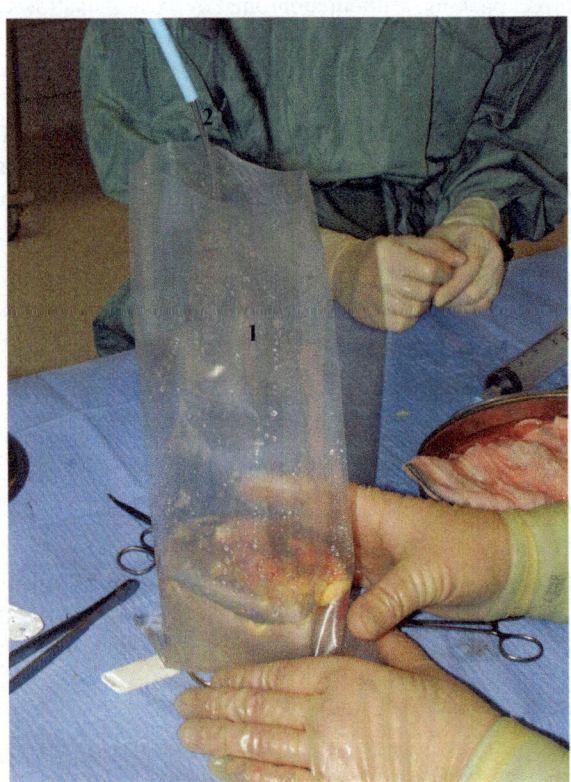

Fig. 17.1 Organ packing. 1 – First bag with procured organ is filled with the preservation solution

17.1 Technique of Organ Packing

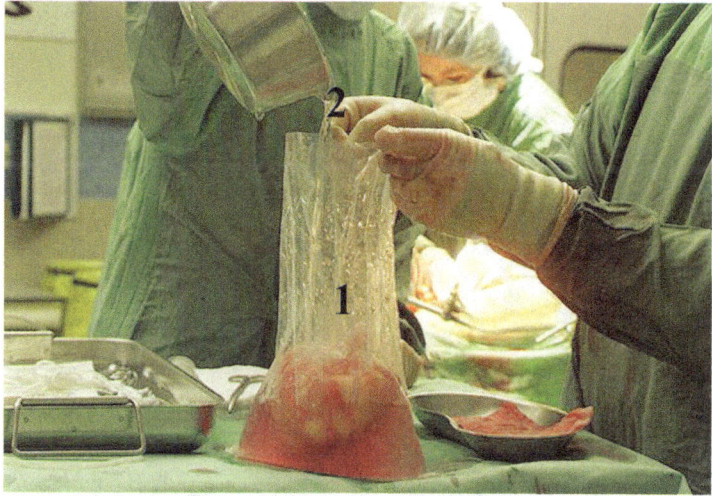

Fig. 17.2 Organ packing. 1 – The second bag is filled with one of the sterile solutions and without air, and is securely tied

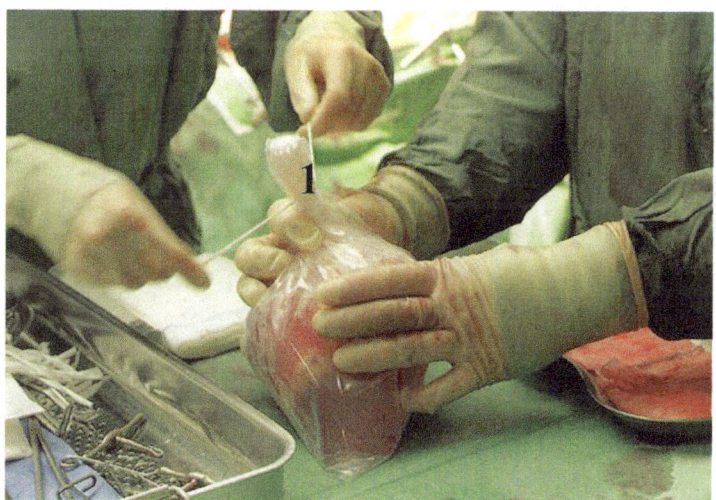

Fig. 17.3 Organ packing. 1 – The third bag is dry, without air and securely tied

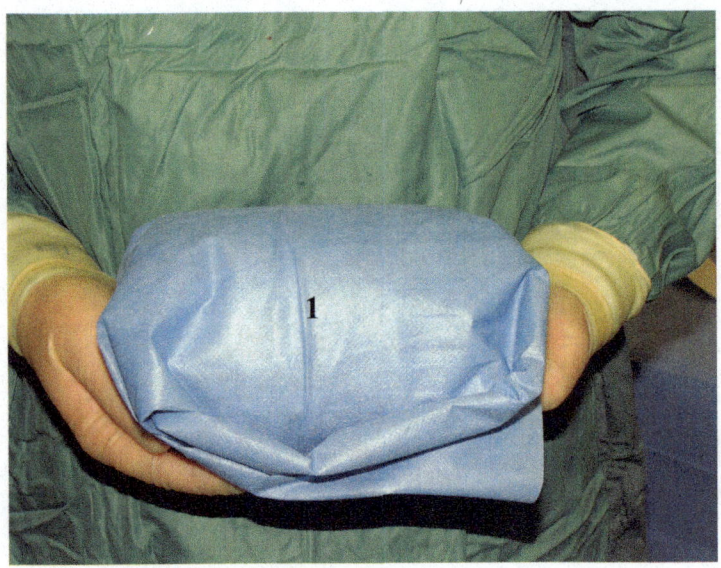

Fig. 17.4 1 – The procured organ is packed in three bags and covered on the back table with a sterile drape

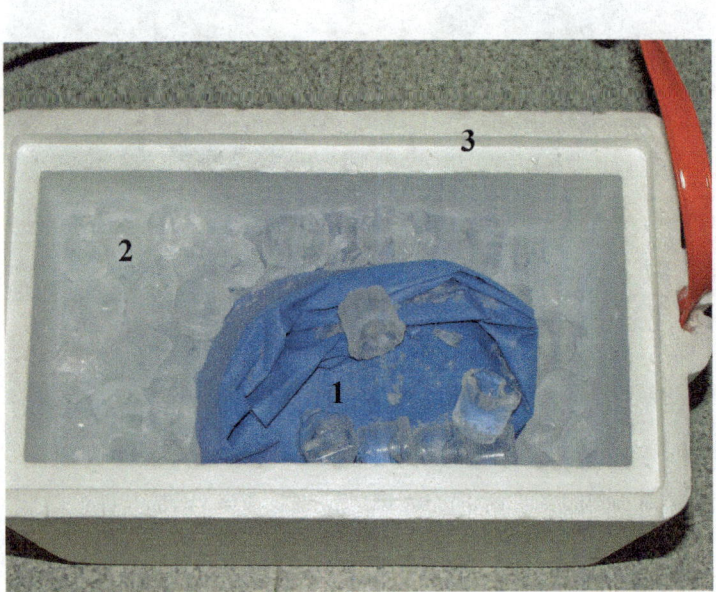

Fig. 17.5 1 – Organ is placed in the transport box on ice and covered with ice. 1 – Procured organ, 2 – Ice, 3 – Transport box

17.1 Technique of Organ Packing

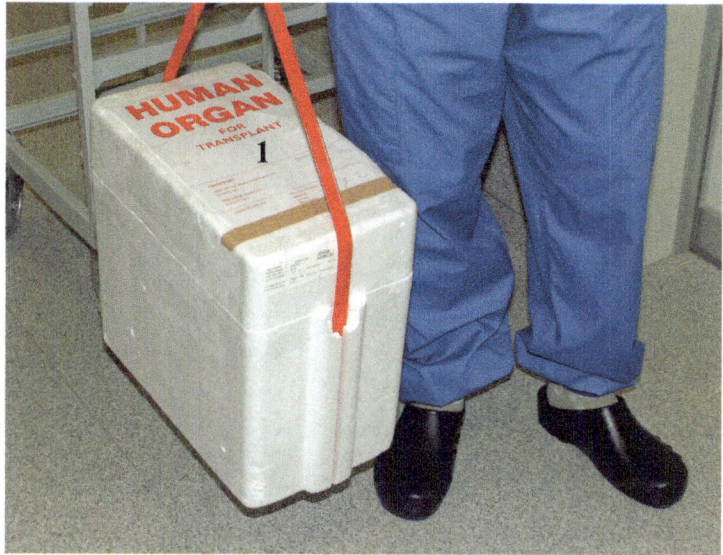

Fig. 17.6 Organ is ready for transportation in the transport box. 1 – Transport box

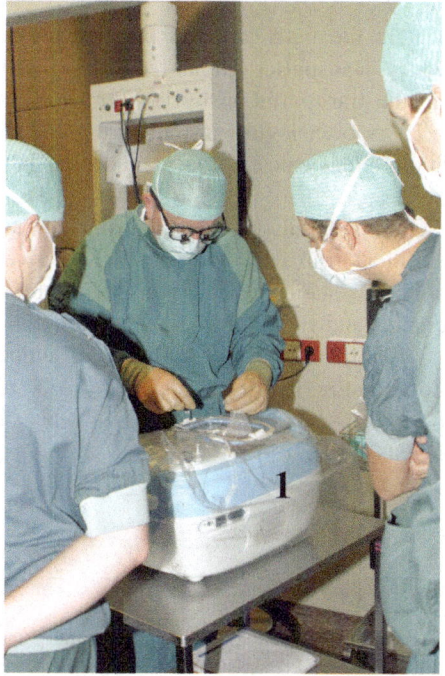

Fig. 17.7 The LifePort Kidney Transporter. 1 – Kidney installation in the mechanical transporter

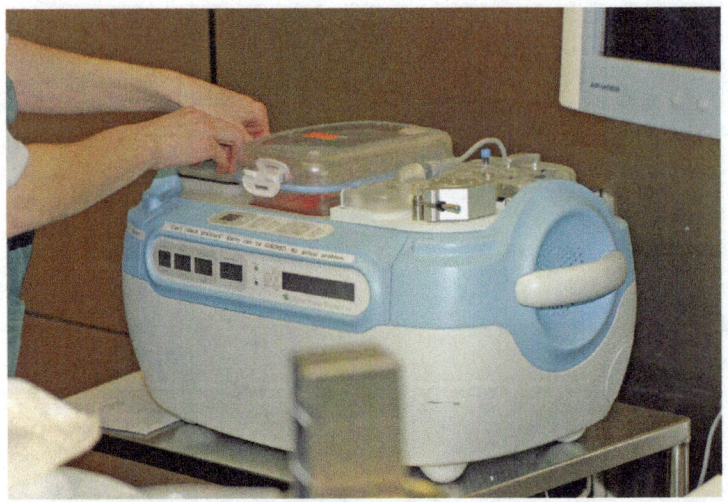

Fig. 17.8 The LifePort Kidney Transporter is almost ready for organ transportation

17.1.3 Kravitz's Lifeport Kidney Transporter

The latest achievement in the field of organ preservation and transportation is Kravitz's LifePort Kidney Transporter (Organ recovery): The first kidney continuously perfused during the transportation by LifePort was transplanted in 2003. The LifePort Kidney Transporter is now in routine use worldwide. LifePort units are now being used in more than a dozen transplant centres in the USA and Europe (Figs. 17.7 and 17.8).

The Machine Preservation Trial (O: PAIRS) group is the first large, international, multi-centre clinical trial to investigate the relative efficacy and cost-effectiveness of machine vs. static preservation. The trial is being conducted in Germany, The Netherlands and Belgium in collaboration with Eurotransplant and the Deutsche Stiftung Organ Transplantation (Started November 1, 2005 and ended November 1, 2006, coordinating PI: Rutger Ploeg, $N = 600$ recipients). In future, small organ transportation machines will be used for other organs such as heart, lung(s), liver and pancreas (1, 2).

Literature

1. Eurotransplant. The Eurotransplant Manual. http//www.eurotransplant.nl
2. Organ Recovery Systems. Machine Preservation Trial. http://www.organ-recovery.com/home.php and/or http://www.organpreservation.nl/

Chapter 18
Post-Procurement Care of the Donor Body

Abstract Background: Closing the donor body is the last surgical step during organ procurement.

The fluid from the thorax and the abdominal cavity is removed. The last inspection of the cavities and remaining organs is done. The body is filled with absorbing materials and closed properly, following the same surgical rules as that followed after every operation. Leakage through the wound after donor closure should be avoided.

Conclusion: Close the donor with great respect for the body, the donor family and so, by definition, respect for yourself.

Keywords Donor body, closing donor, wound dressing

18.1 Before Closing the Donor Body

18.1.1 Surgical Steps

1. Remove residual fluid from the donor body (Fig. 18.1).
2. For the last time examine the remaining organs, the thorax and the abdominal cavity and check for any pathological abnormality.
3. Fill the body with absorbing materials (Fig. 18.2).

18.2 Closing

18.2.1 Surgical Steps

1. Close the thorax and the abdomen with the solid sutures to avoid fluid leakage during transportation and subsequent funeral ceremony (Fig. 18.3).

A. Baranski, *Surgical Technique of the Abdominal Organ Procurement*,
DOI: 10.1007/978-1-84800-251-7_18, © Springer-Verlag London Limited 2009

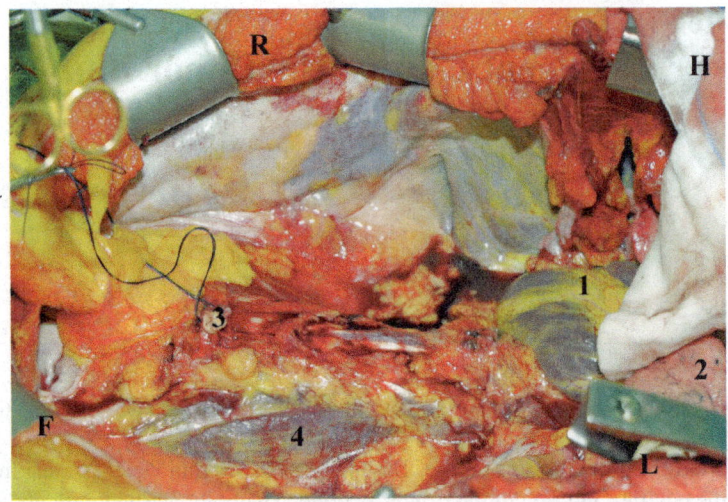

Fig. 18.1 Empty abdominal cavity, residual fluid has been removed. 1 – Non- procured heart, 2 – Non- procured lungs, 3 – Aorta bifurcation, 4 – Psoas major muscle, *H – head, F – feet, R – right, L – left*

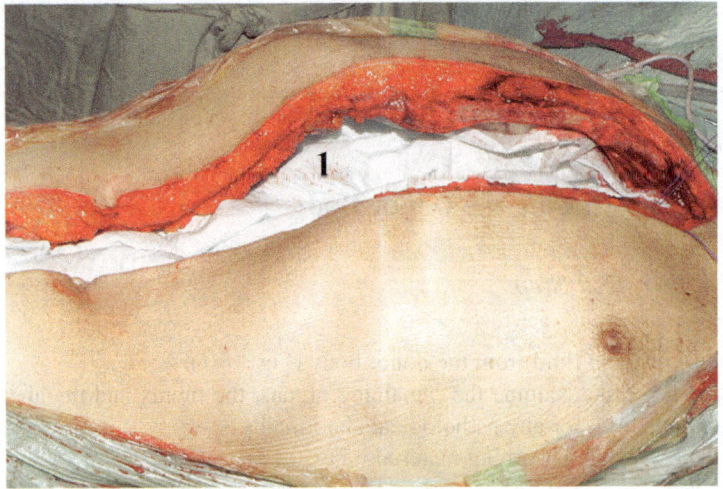

Fig. 18.2 Body cavity filled with absorbing materials

2. Close carefully the midline thoracic incision with interrupted sutures.
3. Close carefully the midline abdominal incision with running sutures.
4. Subcutaneous tissues are closed with a running suture (less chance for liquid leakage, especially if the sternum was not properly closed).
5. Close the skin intracutaneously (Fig. 18.4).

18.2 Closing

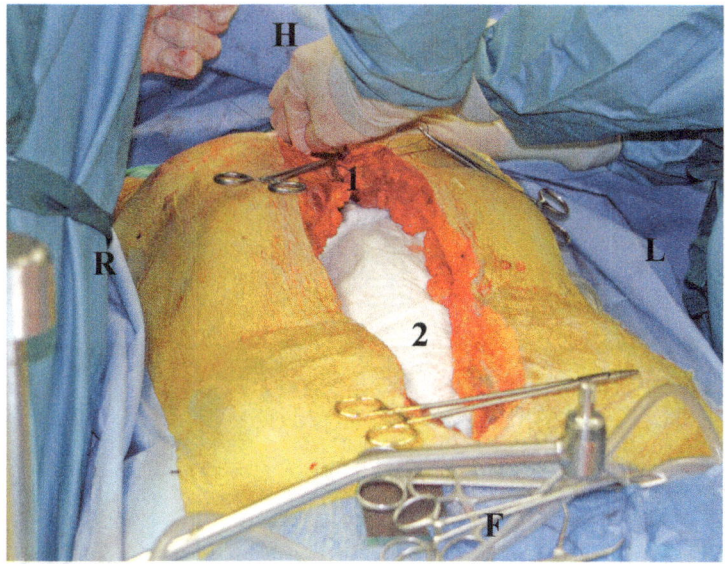

Fig. 18.3 Close 1 – thorax and 2 – abdomen with the solid sutures to avoid fluid leakage

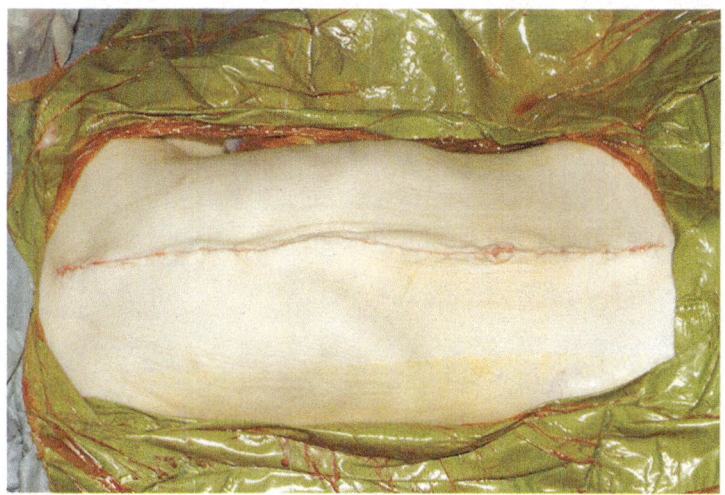

Fig. 18.4 Skin closed intracutaneously

18.2.2 Wound Dressing (Fig. 18.5)

ATTENTION!
Close the donor with great respect for the body, the donor family and so, by definition, respect for yourself.

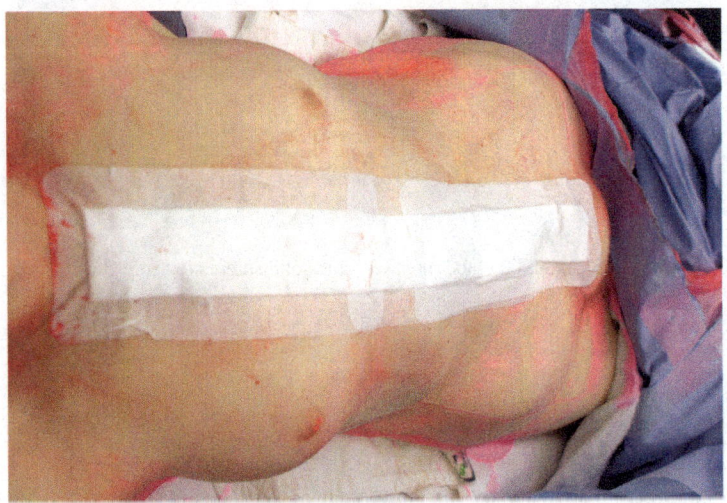

Fig. 18.5 Wound dressing

Chapter 19
Operative Report and the Quality Forms

Abstract Background: By filling the operation report and quality forms, the procurement surgeon fulfils the national or international rules for organ procurement. All findings and decisions that were taken during organ procurement have to be documented. Information must be clear to everybody who was involved in organ procurement and transplantation.

Conclusion: Quality monitoring of procured organs plays an important role in every national transplant program. No technical mistake is the benchmark of a well-trained procurement team with small waiting lists and many successful transplants.

Keywords Operating reports, Quality form, Transplant coordinator, Summary, Oparating room personnel

19.1 Organ Procurement is an Acknowledged Surgical Procedure

19.1.1 Filling Reports

1. Fill in the operation report and quality form, remembering that the signature of the procurement surgeon is mandatory (Figs. 19.1 and 19.2).
2. Filling the operation reports is the confirmation that Eurotransplant or the national organ procurement rules have been fulfilled.
3. A procurement report and completed quality form should be included in the donor protocol.

EUROTRANSPLANT LIVER / PANCREAS REPORT

CENTER: CONTACT TO:

DATE: DONOR Nr: PHONE #:   FAX #:

DONOR IDENTITY:
Date of birth: ...... / ...... / ......   Age: ....yrs   Hospital:
Sex: M / F   Height: .... (cm)   Admission on: ...... / ...... / ...... at .... hrs
                                 Body weight: .... (kg)   Date of death: ...... / ...... / ...... at .... hrs
ABO type: ....   Rhesus: Pos / Neg   Cause of death: ....

HLA-Type: ....
HBs Ag: Pos / Neg   (HBc Ab: Pos / Neg)   HCV Ab: Pos / Neg   HIV Ab: Pos / Neg   CMV IgG: Pos / Neg   (Lues Ab: Pos / Neg)

CLINICAL PARAMETERS (at time of procurement)
Body Temperature: .... °C   Diuresis: .... ml last 24 hrs   **DRUGS**   **dosage**
                                           Last hour: .... ml   Antibiotics: ....
                                                                                   Diuretics: ....
                                                                                    Anti-diuretics: ....
Blood pressure: ....../...... mm Hg   Vasopressors: Dopamine .... µg/kg BW/min
                                        Date /Time   Dobutamine .... µg/kg BW/min
Hypotensive period: Yes / No   ..../........... (Duration: .... min)   Epinephrine .... µg/kg BW/min
Cardiac arrest: Yes / No   ..../........... (Duration: .... min)   Norepinephrine .... µg/kg BW/min
                                                                                                                     Blood transfusions: ....
                                                                                                                     Plasma expanders: ....
                                                                                                                     Other drugs: ....

BIOCHEMISTRY (most recent data)
Urine sediment: Urea: AST: Bilirubin: Hemoglobin: HbA_{1C}:
Urine glucose: Creatinine: ALT: Amylase: Leucocytes: Sputum culture: Pos / Neg
Urine protein: Na^+:   LDH: Lipase: CK: Blood culture: Pos / Neg
Urine culture: Pos / Neg K^+:   γGT: Glucose: CK MB:

PRESERVATION
Heparin: .... IU at .... hrs   Cross clamp time: .... hrs
Cold perfusion Aorta started at .... hrs   Cold perfusion Portal Vein or SMV started at .... hrs
Kind and volume of perfusate: HTK / UW / Other: ....

ANATOMY / EXPLANTATION
LIVER   **PANCREAS**
Normal arterial anatomy: Y / N   Whole / Segmental
If no, specify: With / Without duodenum

Gallbladder flushed   Y / N
Bile duct flushed   Y / N
Coeliac axis: Y / N   Coeliac axis: Y / N
Common hepatic artery: Y / N   Common hepatic artery: Y / N
SMA: Y / N   SMA: Y / N
Aortic patch: Y / N   Aortic patch: Y / N
Portal vein: Long / Short   Portal vein: Long / Short
Cholecystectomy: Y / N
Iliac arteries: Y / N   Iliac arteries: Y / N
Iliac veins: Y / N   Iliac veins: Y / N

QUALITY
LIVER   **PANCREAS**
Perfusion: Good / Acceptable / Poor   Perfusion: Good / Acceptable / Poor
Hepatectomy at: .... hrs   Pancreatectomy at: .... hrs
Reason why liver not used: Reason why pancreas not used:

Quality of liver		Quality of pancreas
Good / Acceptable / Poor		Good / Acceptable / Poor

PROCUREMENT CENTER: PROCUREMENT CENTER:

SURGEON'S NAME ....   SURGEON'S NAME ....

SIGNATURE ....   SIGNATURE ....

Liver transplanted: Y / N   Pancreas transplanted: Y / N

Recipient Center: Recipient Center:

ET Nr: ET Nr:

version dec. 1998

Fig. 19.1 Eurotransplant Foundation's example of liver/pancreas operation report

19.1 Organ Procurement is an Acknowledged Surgical Procedure

PANCREAS QUALITY FORM
to be completed by the surgeon at the time of implantation

Date of Transplant:	__-__-__	Transplant center:	____ P A
Donor Center:	_ T P	Donor number:	____
Procurement Center:	_ T P	Recipient number:	____

Pancreas: **with / without duodenum**

Quality of packaging: ❏ good   ❏ acceptable   ❏ poor

Arterial Problems: [   ]

Venous Problems: [   ]

Duodenal Problems: [   ]

State of Perfusion: ❏ normal   ❏ marbled
Organ report completed: ❏ yes   ❏ no

Quality of Parenchyma: [   ]
(hematoma, injuries)

Duration: Cold ischemia: __ hrs   __ min   Anastomosis: __ min

Reperfusion flow: ❏ normal   ❏ reduced   ❏ none
(if done prior to surgery)

Initial function: ❏ good   ❏ moderate   ❏ bad

Additional remarks/   [   ]
Reason not used:

Name of transplant surgeon: _____   Signature: _____

Please fax to: Please fax to:

MEDICAL STAFF   **PROF. DR:** _____
EUROTRANSPLANT FOUNDATION   **HEAD OF PROCUREMENT – CENTER**
                                         FAX: _____

version sept. 1998

Fig. 19.2 Pancreas quality form – example from Eurotransplant Foundation

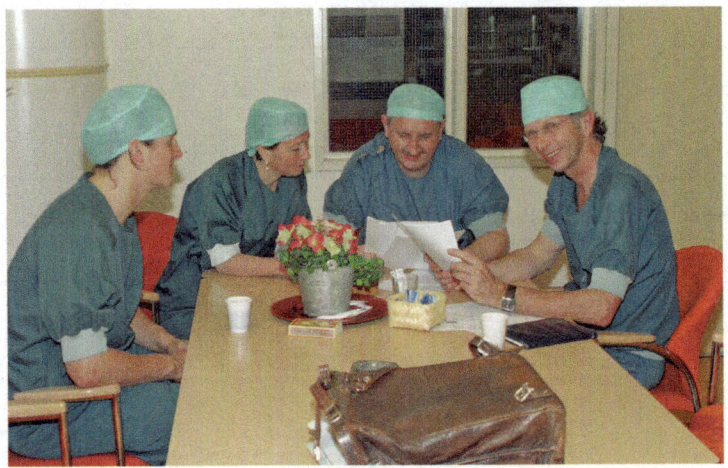

Fig. 19.3 Summation (Debriefing) of the whole procedure

19.1.2 Summation (Debriefing) of the Whole Procedure Together with the OR Personnel and TC (Fig. 19.3)

After every abdominal organ procurement, the surgeon, together with the TC and the hospital personnel involved, have to engage in a short debriefing about the whole procedure. The procurement surgeon has to be the leader in this discussion and guide it pleasantly through all the relevant stages: what went well, what went wrong, and what could be done to improve the procedure next time. The communication skills of the procurement surgeon are as important as his other abilities because a successful debriefing, which achieves the goals and does not offend anyone, will ensure continued (or improved) cooperation between the two teams at each subsequent meeting.

Index

A
Abdominal aorta
  and IVC, ligation and cannulation
    of, 104–109
  perfusion system, 99–101 (*see also* Organ
    perfusion, preparation of)
  surgical procedures in, 55–63
  visualisation of, 72–74
Abdominal incision, 21–26
Abdominal organ perfusion, 113–114
  to check efficiency of system, 116–117
  clamp removal, 114–115
  topical cooling, 115–116
Abdominal organ procurement
  abdominal dissection of
    Cattel–Braasch manoeuvre, 45–53
    infrarenal and SMA, major vessel
      dissection, 55–64
  abdominal organ protection, 93–96
  abdominal organs, inspection of
    gut, 43
    liver, 34–39
    pancreas, 39–43
  communication in (*see* Communication)
  donor coordinator services, 2–3
  left liver lobe mobilisation in, 66–72
  preoperative arrangements of
    abdominal procurement team arrival,
      9–12
    abdominal retractor installation, 19–20
    donor verification, 12–13
    draping of donor, 17–19
    positioning of donor, 13–14
    scrubbing of donor, 15–17
    shaving of donor, 14–15
  right liver lobe mobilisation, surgical
    procedures of, 74
  sequence of, 120–123
  small bowel procurement, 89
  wide, stable operating field in
    abdominal and thorax retractor,
      30–32
    abdominal incision, 21–26
    median sternotomy, 26–30
Abdominal organ protection, 93–96
Abdominal organ transplantation, donor
  criteria in, xv
Abdominal retractor, 19–20, 30, 51, 67, 104
Abdominal vessel cannulation
  abdominal aorta and IVC, ligation and,
    104–109
  agreement in, 103–104
Aberrant hepatic artery, 37–39, 42, 70–72, 77,
  78, 132, 135, 147, 148
  anatomy of, 84
Amphotericin B, 129, 130
Aorta's perfusion system, 99

B
Blumhardt, G., 168
Brockman, J. G., 117

C
Cattel–Braasch manoeuvre, 45–46, 52
Cholecystectomy, 81, 167, 168
Chui, A. K., 117
Cirrhosis, 35
Cold perfusion, 127
  start abdominal organ perfusion,
    113–114
  clamp removal, 114–115
  efficiency of, 116–117
  topical cooling, 115–116
  start thoracic organ perfusion, 111–112
Colledan, M., 117
Colon, physiological positioning of, 65–66

Common bile duct (CBD), 75, 84, 85, 87, 144, 148, 159
    dissection, surgical procedures for, 79–81
Communication
    before cannulation, OR personnel, 103
    skills, 1, 2, 7, 103
    between TC and surgeon
        after organ procurement, 6–7
        before organ procurement, 3–5
        during organ procurement, 5–6

D
de Ville de Goyet, J., 117
Donor body
    closing the
        surgical steps, 195–198
        wound dressing, 198
    post-procurement care of
        before closing the, 195
    warming, to avoid coagulation, 16
Donor coordinator services, organ procurement, 2–3
Donor preoperative arrangements, 9–12
Donor scrubbing, 16
Donor shaving, 14–15
Donor verification, 12
Draping, 17, 18
Duodenopancreatic mobilisation, surgical steps for, 48–50

E
Edema, 35
Electrocautery, 21, 23, 26, 29, 31, 46, 67, 68, 70, 72
European Donor Surgery Masterclass (EDSM), xvi
European Society for Organ Transplantation (ESOT), xvi
Eurotransplant and the Deutsche Stiftung Organ Transplantation, 194
Eurotransplant Foundation, 200, 201
Eurotransplant regulations, for organ packing, 189
Extended Kocher manoeuvre, 42
    in duodenopancreatic mobilisation, 46, 48–50

F
Fibrosis, 35
Filipponi, F., 117
Florman, S. S., 119
Freed supraceliac abdominal aorta, 74

G
Gabel, M., 117
Gall bladder, dissection of, 81–83
Gastrocolic ligament, 39, 40, 90, 132, 133
Gastroduodenal dissection, surgical procedures of, 84–86
Gastrointestinal stapling device (GIA), 90, 126, 128, 130, 131, 138, 140
General cleanliness and readiness, 10
Gudykunst, W. B., 6
Gut inspection, 43

H
Heart-beating donor (HBD), 3, 101, xv
Heparinization, 7, 63, 95
Hepatic artery, surgical procedures of, 84–86
Hepatoduodenal ligament, 38, 75–76
    inspection of, 76–78
Hepatogastric ligament, 36, 39, 40, 67, 70, 72, 75
Histidine-tryptophan-ketoglutarate (HTK), 97–99

I
Iaria, G., 117
Iliac veins, in tool-kit, 185
Inferior mesenteric artery (IMA), 45, 53, 58, 59, 61, 62
Inferior mesenteric vein (IMV), 45, 53, 55, 56, 58, 103
Inferior part of sternotomy, 24
Inferior vena cava (IVC), 42, 45, 47, 49, 52, 76, 162
    bisected IVC above diaphragm, 163
    bisected IVC below liver, 170
    bisected left renal vein from, 160
    cutting totally, helpful during decompression, 117
    decompression system, preparation technique, 101–102
    divided IVC, 161
    fixed with clamp IVC ligature, 112
    fourth finger in, 165
    index finger in the, 166
    ligation and cannulation, surgical steps, 104–109
    surgical procedures in, 55–63
Infrarenal dissection, 55
Intensive care unit (ICU), 2, 12, 13
Islets of Langergans, 159
IVC decompression system, 101–102. *See also* Organ perfusion, preparation of

Index

J
Jejunum, 90, 126–128

K
Kidney procurement
  aorta and IVC cannulas, removal of, 170
  aorta anterior side opening, 171
  aorta bisected above bifurcation and splitting, 172
  cutting abdominal aorta, above bifurcation, 169
  cutting aortic patch, for left kidney, 174
  cutting IVC, above its bifurcation, 169, 172
  cutting ligatures, 169
  en block kidney procurement, 178–180
    renal vessels, examination of, 179
  kidney mobilisation, 173
  mobilising, the right kidney aorta patch, 174
  reducing fat around kidney, 178
  separation of kidneys, procured en block in steps, 180–183
Kocher manoeuver, 41. *See also* Extended Kocher manoeuvre
Komokata, T., 117
Kravitz's LifePort Kidney Transporter, 189, 194

L
Left liver lobe mobilisation, surgical procedures of, 66–72
Leiden University Medical Centre, xvi
Ligament inspection, and dissection, 75–78
Ligation and cannulation, of abdominal aorta, 104–109
Lingard, L., 6
Liver arterial blood supply, examination of, 35–39
Liver inspection, 34–39
  before transplantation, 121
Liver procurement
  cholecystectomy, with cystic duct ligation, 167
  cutting from IVC patch, with left renal vein, 159
  cutting left leaflet, of diaphragm, 162, 164
  dividing IVC between liver and kidneys, 161–162
  en block procurement–indications, 168–169
  ostium of right renal vein, 161
  pericardium, after heart procurement, 163
  puttiing forefinger in IVC, 162–164, 166
  right diaphragm, not try to dissect, 162, 164

Liver, protected by wet large gauze, 25
Liver steatosis, 35
  open biopsy, 43
Lung inspection, 32

M
Machine Preservation Trial (O: PAIRS) group, 194
Macrovesical steatosis, 35
Marino, I. R, 117
Median laparotomy, 22, 25
Median sternotomy, 26–30
Mesenteric vessels, 90, 126
Microvesicular steatosis, 35
Mizrahi, S. S., 169
Moench, C., 168
Multi-organ donation, procedure, 7

N
National Courses on the Abdominal Multi Organ Donation, xvi
National Dutch Transplant Foundation, xvi
National Transplant Organization, 189
Necessary surgical equipment, 11
Non-heart-beating donor (NHBD), 3
Normal liver arterial blood supply (NLABS), 37

O
Oesophagus, dissected, 73
Omni Track®, 20
Operating room (OR), 4, 9
Organ assessment, in pancreas inspection, 42–43
Organ dissection, 32, 125, xv
Organ donation, 2, 35
Organ inspection, 33–35
  investigations during, 43
Organ packing, technique of, 189–194
Organ perfusion, preparation of
  abdominal aorta perfusion system, 99–101
  IVC decompression system, 101–102
  preservation solution for, 97–99
Organ procurement
  debriefing, OR personnel and TC, 202
  filling operation reports and quality form, 199–202
    liver/pancreas operation report, 200
    pancreas quality form, 201
  organization, 2
Organ retrieval team(s), 1

Organ transplantation, 1, 7, 149, 157
    process, tool-kit role in, 185–188

P

Pancreas and liver vascular splitting
    advantages of, splitting liver
        and pancreas, 149
    cutting gastroduodenal artery, 143
    cutting portal vein and splenic artery, 143
    cutting SMA with aortic patch, 156–157
        from aorta with patch, 157
        celiac plexus dissection, 156
    dissecting common hepatic artery, 143
    dorsal pancreatic artery, arising from
        common hepatic artery, 147
    hepatoduodenal ligament, vascular
        dissection of, 143
    intra-pancreatic course, of right aberrant
        hepatic artery, 147
    pancreas procured with celiac trunk and,
        148 (see also Pancreas
        procurement)
    in presence of right aberrant hepatic
        artery, 147
    stump of gastroduodenal artery, 144
    vascular arterial splitting, possibilities
        of, 149
    whole pancreas procurement, for islets
        isolation, 157–159
Pancreas arterial reconstruction, with aortic
    arch, 186
Pancreas head mobilisation, 46, 49
Pancreas inspection, 39–43
Pancreas, liver, kidneys, procurement surgical
    technique, 126
    closing duodenum at level of pyrolus, 131
    dividing duodenum
        from jejunum, 128
        from stomach, 130
    povidone iodine and amphotericin B,
        injection, 129–130
    pylorus and Treitz ligament, marking
        of level, 127
    replacing gastric tube, 128–129
    small bowel and colon, placing outside
        abdomen, 136–142
    sterilizing duodenum content, 128
    stomach mobilisation, 132–135
    stomach tube, replaced to duodenum, 129
Pancreas procurement, 149
    cutting spleen for laboratory typing, 154
    high risk, of pancreas tail damage, 154
    spleen and pancreas, tail mobilisation,
        149–155
    splenectomy, during back-table process, 155
    for whole organ transplantation, 149
Pancreas quality form, 201
Parenchyma inspection, in liver, 35–36
Ploeg, R., 194
Portal vein dissection, surgical steps
    for, 86–87
Positioning donor, on operating table, 13
Povidone iodine, 129
Preservation solution, 97–99
Previous laparotomy scars(s), 23
Procurement surgeon, duties of, 5–6

R

Rapid perfusion system, 100
Right aberrant hepatic artery. See Aberrant
    hepatic artery
Right colon mobilisation, surgical steps for,
    46–47
Right liver lobe mobilisation, surgical
    steps in, 74
Ringer lactate, 115, 126, 157, 166, 175, 190

S

Scrubbing. See Donor scrubbing
Shaving. See Donor shaving
Small bowel
    dissection, surgical procedures of, 90
    mobilisation, surgical steps in, 51–53
    physiological positioning of, 65–66
    procurement of, 89, 126
Start median sternotomy, 26
Steatosis, 35
Sterile post, 19
Sternotomy with Gigli's saw, 28
Superior mesenteric artery (SMA), 37, 39, 45,
    46, 49, 148, 152, 156, 183, 186
    dissected SMA, 63
    ligate and cut small branches of, 90, 126
    surgical procedures for, 64
Supraceliac aorta, 65, 113, 153
Surgical access routes, in pancreas, 39–42

T

Thompson®, 20
Thompson professional abdominal retractor, 18
Thoracic organ perfusion, 111–113
Thoracic organ procurement, 119–120
    for abdominal organ, sequence of, 120–123
    procurement
        disease of thoracic wall, 123
        heart before packing, 120

    internal and external cooling during, 123
    lungs before packing, 122
Thoracic organs dissection, 95
Thorax procurement team, 95–96
Thorax retractor, 30–32
Tisone, G., 117
Tokunaga, Y., 117
Tool-kit
    in organ transplantation process, 185–188
    packing, 188
    procurement–iliac arteries, 187
Transplant coordinator (TC), 1–7
Transport box, 192–193
Treitz ligament, 50, 51, 126–128, 137

U
University of Winsconsin (UW) solution, 98

V
Van Damme, J. P., 36

W
White line of Toldt, 45, 47

Y
Yersiz, H., 89

Made in the USA
Monee, IL
03 May 2026